Clinical Supervision: Theory and Practice

Clinical Supervision: Theory and Practice

LORI A. RUSSELL-CHAPIN
Bradley University
WITH
THEODORE J. CHAPIN

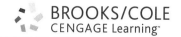

BROOKS/COLE
CENGAGE Learning™

Australia • Brazil • Japan • Korea • Mexico • Singapore • Spain • United Kingdom • United States

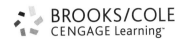

BROOKS/COLE
CENGAGE Learning™

Clinical Supervision: Theory and Practice
Lori A. Russell-Chapin with Theodore J. Chapin

Acquisitions Editor: Seth Dobrin

Assistant Editor: Alicia Mclaughlin

Editorial Assistant: Suzanna Kincaid

Media Editor: Elizabeth Momb

Marketing Assistant: Gurpreet Saran

Marketing Communications Manager: Tami Strang

Content Project Manager: Rita Jaramillo

Design Director: Rob Hugel

Art Director: Caryl Gorska

Print Buyer: Linda Hsu

Rights Acquisitions Specialist: Don Schlotman

Production Service: MPS Limited, a Macmillan Company

Copy Editor: Jill Pellarin

Cover Design and iconography: Angie Wang and Mark Fox, Design is Play

Compositor: MPS Limited, a Macmillan Company

© 2012 Brooks/Cole, Cengage Learning

For product information and technology assistance, contact us at
Cengage Learning Customer & Sales Support, 1-800-354-9706

For permission to use material from this text or product, submit all requests online at **www.cengage.com/permissions**
Further permissions questions can be e-mailed to
permissionrequest@cengage.com

Library of Congress Control Number: 2010928365

Student Edition:
ISBN-13: 978-0-495-00915-3
ISBN-10: 0-495-00915-6

Brooks/Cole
20 Davis Drive
Belmont, CA 94002-3098USA

Cengage Learning is a leading provider of customized learning solutions with office locations around the globe, including Singapore, the United Kingdom, Australia, Mexico, Brazil, and Japan. Locate your local office at: **www.cengage.com/global.**

Cengage Learning products are represented in Canada by Nelson Education, Ltd.

To learn more about BrooksCole, visit **www.cengage.com/brookscole**

Purchase any of our products at your local college store or at our preferred online store **www.cengagebrain.com.**

Printed in the United States of America
1 2 3 4 5 6 7 14 13 12 11 10

Table of Contents

Chapter 4 Developmental Supervision Models   47

Chapter 5 Theoretical Specific Supervision Models   65

Chapter 6 Social Role Supervision Models   87

Chapter 9 Realizing the Many Benefits of Group Supervision   135

Chapter 10 Future Directions in Supervision   173

About the Authors

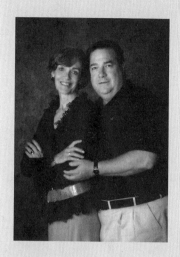

Dr. Lori Russell-Chapin was the Chair of the graduate counseling program for 11 years at Bradley University in Peoria, Illinois. Currently, she is a Professor and the Associate Dean of the College of Education and Health Sciences at Bradley. She continues to teach practicum and internship, crisis intervention, introduction to the profession, and ethics courses. She works in private practice with her husband, Ted, and has worked as a clinical supervisor for many years. She is a Licensed Clinical Professional Counselor, an NBCC Approved Clinical Supervisor and a Certified Clinical Mental Health Counselor. Lori is an award-winning teacher at Bradley with numerous peer-reviewed journal publications, books, and creative productions. She and Dr. Allen Ivey are the coauthors of *Your Supervised Practicum and Internship: Field Resources for Turning Theory into Practice.*

Dr. Ted Chapin has been the President of Resource Management Services, a comprehensive consultation and employee assistance program, and Chapin & Russell Associates, a counseling private practice, for the past 20 years in Peoria, Illinois. He teaches at Bradley University on a part-time basis as needed. He is a licensed clinical psychologist and marriage and family therapist.

Preface

The Beginnings of This Supervision Text

This supervision book has taken on a life of its own. The reasons are numerous. The first occurred when a master counselor came to one of the textbook's authors, Lori, for supervision, with a look of total puzzlement on his face. His name was Bryan, and he began supervision before Lori could even ask, "What would you like to work on in supervision today?" He was shaking his head and exclaiming, "I don't know what to do with this fairly healthy client! For years I have been working with mostly chemically addicted male clients. Now I have a female, nonaddicted person who talks a lot, and I think I am lost in counseling. I haven't been lost in a long time."

Bryan showed Lori his tape, and the genesis for this book began. Lori realized then that the manner in which she had been doing supervision was effective and efficient for Bryan's male addicted clients, but it would not work for this client.

Bryan was kind enough, flexible enough, and confused enough to experiment with differing supervision styles. He and his client courageously consented to using one of their supervision sessions so Lori could demonstrate five different supervision approaches. In the end, Bryan was asked which approach met his and his client's supervision needs the most. His answer was surprising yet understandable. What Bryan needed was not the typical cognitive behavioral supervision session. His confidence had been tested with a new population. He was questioning many of his solid addiction counseling skills. Lori used all five supervision models with his same supervision question: "What am I doing wrong? She just keeps talking and I don't feel connected. I want to get her into process but it is too difficult."

Bryan discussed the benefits of each supervision model, but the approach that seemed to help Bryan the most this time and responded best to his need and supervision question was theoretic specific. By modeling back during this supervision session, a variation of an Empty Chair technique that Bryan tried to use with his client, Bryan realized that his skills can generalize from population to population and that he needed to relax. Bryan also concluded that supervision over the life span of a counseling career can keep helping professionals sharp and less stressed. Bryan and Lori's videotaping experience was the genesis for this book; it seemed natural to expand on this idea and format.

Another reason for this type of supervision book is that both authors, Lori and Ted, practice counseling privately in a group practice. Lori teaches full time at a private, midwestern university, Bradley University, and is able to consult 8 hours per week at their private practice. The supervision needs of private practitioners, agency and school counselors, and graduate students differ, but the need for a supervision book for all settings seemed apparent.

The Benefits and Purpose of This Text

Therefore, this supervision textbook will provide a "one-stop shopping" approach for all users whereby the reader can review supervision theory, discover individual supervision style, read about five supervision approaches to clinical supervision, observe a demonstration of those approaches, and watch an agency group supervision in action. The demonstrations can be accessed through the packaged DVD included with the book. The demonstrations will not show *the* way to conduct supervision, but they will show the authors' interpretation and style of the clinical supervision approaches and group supervision. In the individual supervision sessions, Lori is the supervisor. In the group supervision session, Lori is the supervisee and Ted is the supervisor.

In the world of clinical supervision, there are excellent supervision resources explaining academic theory and skills. However, it became clear that there were several missing pieces in the supervision knowledge base. Nowhere were there demonstrations and hands-on materials to which supervisors, supervisees, and/or students from different settings could turn when they were lost in the supervisory therapeutic process. Nowhere was there a resource that could actually demonstrate the differing styles and approaches to clinical supervision. There are many wonderful books and manuals on supervision, but nowhere was there one resource where all this information was integrated in a comprehensive manner.

This textbook will also focus on individual and group supervision and offer a strong knowledge base about supervision. The information gained will aid supervisees and supervisors in growing at a faster pace and becoming more autonomous in their developmental journey as helping professionals. Additionally, supervision approaches that will assist the reader in becoming more versatile, knowledgeable, and flexible will be explored. The approaches are developed from unique philosophical frameworks underlying the supervision process. Practical examples from each approach will be offered.

Textbook Outcomes

The reader may also follow along with the DVD using transcripts from the supervisor and supervisee located in the corresponding chapters. A demonstration of typical community/agency group supervision can also be accessed through the DVD. In addition, each chapter will offer reflective exercises so the supervisor and supervisee can practice and expand and integrate supervision outcomes.

By the time the reader reaches the end of this book, he or she will be able to answer these questions: What do I need from supervision? What is my supervision style? Why should supervision continue over the lifespan of a counseling career? How can a supervisor minimize some of the potentially harmful effects of psychological treatment for a supervisee? Many additional questions will be answered as well. Each chapter has several reflection questions offered throughout the chapter topics. The more questions the reader is willing to complete, the more supervision information can be gleaned from each important supervision chapter.

Supervision Chapter Topics

The authors believe that the topics in each chapter are critical to the success of the supervisory process. In these chapters are direct and practical applications for the supervisee and the supervisor. **Chapter One, *A Clarifying View of Supervision,*** defines clinical counseling supervision and encourages helping professionals to see the overall benefits of supervision throughout the life span of the counseling career. The basic tenets and definitions correlate with the roles, qualities, expectations, and functions of the supervisor/supervisee. A supervision policy is presented as an essential component of a supervisory team.

Chapter Two, *Obstacles to Effective Supervision,* offers the optimal combination of four important supervisory factors. These factors include the supervisee, supervisor, the supervisory relationship, and the structural elements of supervision. This chapter explores each of these factors and the potential obstacles they present for effective supervision, and offers some suggestions on how these obstacles can either be avoided or appropriately managed should they arise. The importance of understanding potentially harmful effects of treatment is also emphasized.

In **Chapter Three, *Ethics in Counseling Supervision,*** the entire focus is on the ethical practice of clinical supervision. Each section presents an ethical problem that could readily arise in any setting where mental health services are provided. The reader is presented the problem with a set of discussion questions encouraging further reflection on the particular ethical dilemma. A short summary of the relevant ethical guidelines is provided, followed by a suggested course of appropriate action.

Chapter Four, *Developmental Supervision Models,* is the first of five chapters devoted to differing supervision models. The discussion begins by offering a common-factor approach to supervision, identifying common elements throughout all supervision models. The chapter then provides an overview of developmental models of supervision. Each of the supervision model chapters is formatted describing the **Basic Tenets, When to Use, Supervisor's Emphasis and Goals, Supervisee Growth Areas,** and **Limitations.** This chapter has the transcript and DVD supervision session, The Case of Brad, demonstrating the Stoltenberg, McNeil, and Delworth developmental supervision model. Brad is a master-level social worker with 25 years of counseling experience. His supervision question was "When my client sabotages the counseling outcome, what additional strategies could I implement?"

Theoretical Specific Supervision Models is the title for **Chapter Five.** This chapter focuses on the advantages and disadvantages of using theoretical specific supervision models. The five different psychotherapy-based supervision models highlighted are Rogerian, Rational Emotive Therapy, psychodynamic, attachment, and feminist supervision models. Each model is formatted with the same constructs of **Basic Tenets, When to Use, Supervisor's Emphasis and Goals, Supervisee Growth Areas,** and **Limitations.** Again the transcription is included in this chapter for the DVD demonstration using a psychodynamic supervision model and The Case of Julie. In this DVD segment, Julie is an internship student about ready to graduate with a Master's in Counseling. Her supervision question was "How can I best approach my client's invitation to hear him sing at the Battle of the Bands?"

Chapter Six, *Social Role Supervision Models,* provides the benefit of identifying and emphasizing the varied roles and foci that supervisors need. These supervision models offer structure and interventions for both the supervisee and supervisor. The models also assist the supervisory process by emphasizing the importance of interpersonal communication skills used by the supervisee. Bernard's Discrimination Supervision Model, Holloway's Social Role Supervision Model, and Hawkins and Shohet's Social Role Supervision Model showcase this type of supervision, using the same format as in the above chapters.

The DVD supervision demonstration in this chapter utilizes the discrimination supervision model in THE CASE OF KEVIN. This relatively new counselor is a first-tiered, licensed, master-level counselor. Kevin's supervision question was "My client has switched coping mechanisms from cutting to tattooing. Now she wants even healthier coping strategies. How can I assist her in moving in that direction?" To follow along when viewing the DVD, there is a transcript of the entire session.

In **Chapter Seven,** *Integrated Models of Supervision,* the supervision models tend to be atheoretical and use concepts from other counseling theories that are needed by supervisees. Integrated supervision models are designed for those who work from multiple theoretical orientations. Two approaches toward developing an integrated model are technical eclecticism and theoretical integration.

In this chapter the integrated model of microcounseling supervision (MSM) uses the same written format as previous chapters. MSM utilizes both technical eclecticism and theoretical integration. This model introduces a standardized approach to supervision offering the supervisee strengths and areas for improvement. The Counseling Interview Rating Form (CIRF) is the instrument created for assessment. Follow along using the chapter transcription for a demonstration of the microcounseling supervision model, an integrated and competency-based supervision model, in THE CASE OF CATE. Her supervisee's questions were twofold: "Susan seems to be doing well in this stage of sobriety. Could you give some guidelines as to when to push and when to back off? Once I get to process-oriented material, what do I do?"

Cate is a nontraditional graduate student who already has a PhD in Communications and is changing career fields. She is in a master's practicum counseling course seeing clients for the first time.

Interpersonal Process Recall in **Chapter Eight** creates an example of a widely used supervision approach developed by Norm Kagan. When supervision sessions require videotaping of counseling interviews or conducting counseling sessions in an actual live observation setting, interpersonal process recall (IPR) can be utilized. This supervision approach allows supervisees to safely analyze their thoughts and feelings about the counseling interview. The chapter is written in the same format as the above chapters, providing suggestions of possible supervisory IPR leads and questions.

Transcripts are provided for the DVD demonstration illustrating IPR in THE CASE OF CHAKA. This supervisee is a master-level prepared high school counselor working with a large and diverse school population. She is completing her first year as a high school counselor and is a National Certified Counselor and waiting for her license as a professional counselor. Chaka's supervisory question was "How can I become more effective and clear in my lead, open-ended questions? Lack of clarity often makes me feel less confident and secure in my counseling direction."

Chapter Nine, *Realizing the Benefits of Group Supervision,* outlines the purpose, the advantages of group supervision, and some limitations of this supervision model. It will also delineate a procedure that can be readily applied to many mental health settings. Special attention will be given to the facilitator's role and the many clinical issues that group supervision session can address. The chapter closes with a brief review of some related but vitally important topics that will explore some of the following questions: Should participation in group supervision be voluntary or mandatory? Should mental health professional be charged for supervision? What kind of documentation will the facilitator need to keep? How can a group handle an issue involving an impaired therapist? How does group supervision change in various work settings? When is group supervision just not enough?

The Group Supervision DVD demonstrates a typical bimonthly multidisciplinary, private practice supervision session where there is a designated supervisor and supervisees. However, just like group counseling, the focus on the supervisor changes, and the supervisees become an active part of the supervisory process and team. There are three unique cases presented during this session, ranging from grief and loss, to alcohol treatment, to post traumatic stress. Each supervisee has a distinct supervision question. In this group session, Lori, who has been the supervisor in all the individual supervision demonstrations, is now a supervisee. A transcript of the supervision session is included.

The final chapter is designed to bring closure to the supervision textbook by discussing numerous variables and new directions impacting the field of counseling supervision. **Chapter Ten,** *Future Directions in Supervision,* divides the chapter into 10 distinct topics that may influence the future. The topics range from technology to brain research to gerontology to evidenced-based and competency-based practices. The need for a Professional Supervision Will is also discussed, and a sample is offered.

Following Chapter Ten are the **Appendices.** Appendix A provides the reader with blank forms to be used during the internship, and Appendix B lists several online sources for information on professional organizations and codes of ethics. Appendix C shows a blank Counseling Interview Rating Form (CIRF) from Chapter 7. Appendix D lists a glossary of the 43 skills used in the CIRF. In Appendix E are five additional practice case studies for supervisees and supervisors to test their knowledge of the different supervision models. The cases represent a wide variety of presenting concerns. Case Study 1 reports a 27-year-old female who is dealing with independence issues and mild depression. Case Study 2 is a 42-year-old male struggling with the suicide of his wife. Case Study 3 is a 68-year-old female working with her bipolar diagnosis. Case Study 4 is a 20-year-old male reacting to sleep-related issues and poor decision-making skills. Case Study 5 presents a 38-year-old female who was referred to counseling by her boss because of work-related concerns.

Read through each case presentation. They are formatted using a case presentation standardized guide complete with a DSM-IV-TR diagnosis. Analyze the supervisory question with the case information. Select the "best fit" model for each situation. At the end of each case are several discussion questions to assist you in decision making. Use only one "best fit" model from the five supervision models presented in the chapters. The authors' preferred choices are presented in Appendix F.

The Supervision Journey

Every year I ask each of my new graduate students this question: Did you choose the counseling profession or did the counseling profession choose you? It is a wonderful reflection question, and somewhere, I am sure, the answer lies in the middle of the continuum. The supervision journey has a different answer, however. Each of us in the counseling profession can choose supervision as a lifelong aspect of our counseling career.

I so enjoy being a trained and certified supervisor, but I thrive as a counselor, professor, and supervisor when I am the recipient of continued supervision. As I change and grow in my counseling skill level, so do my supervision needs. Even after all these years, I need and want continued supervision. My supervision journey continues to expand and become more complex. Therefore, regular supervision leaves me rejuvenated, wiser, and healthier. The following quote helps me better understand the need for supervision, for I know that each of us, whether a client, student, colleague, or counselor, has a special yearning for competency. Become a believer in lifelong supervision and observe what happens to your counseling and supervision skill set!

Every blade of grass has its Angel bending over and whispering, "Grow, grow."—The Talmud

Acknowledgements

This book is dedicated to all of our supervisors who taught us compassionately how to counsel, teach, consult, and behave in a professional manner. Thank you for your wisdom. Your guidance and support makes a world of difference.

We would also like to thank the following persons who assisted us in reviewing this book in its manuscript form: Jill Pellarin and Lindsay Schmonsees. A special thank you to the editorial staff at Brooks/Cole/Cengage Learning and especially to Seth Dobrin, our main editor, whose skills and dedication made this textbook a reality.

A Clarifying View of Supervision

Supervision Defined

Much like counseling theories, supervision approaches have many similarities and differences. Most supervision models/approaches emphasize the importance of a healthy supervisee and supervisor relationship, stress the importance of feedback and communication, and have a variety of supervisor tasks and functions. With that in mind, supervision is often defined concisely as a distinctive approach and response to a supervisee's needs from an expert who has more experience (Russell-Chapin & Ivey, 2004; Bernard & Goodyear, 2008). Haynes, Corey, and Moulton (2003) add that clinical supervision is a process using consistent observation and evaluation from a trained counseling professional who has a specialized body of knowledge and skill. Bernard and Goodyear (2004) offer this definition:

> Supervision is an intervention provided by a senior member of a profession to a junior member or members of that same profession. This relationship is: evaluative, extends over time and has the simultaneous purposes of enhancing the professional functioning of the more junior person(s), monitoring the quality of professional services offered to clients that she, he or they see(s), and serving as a gatekeeper of those who are to enter a particular profession (p. 8).

Discussion Questions 1

1. What is your definition of supervision? _____

_____

_____

_____

_____

2. What do you believe the benefits of supervision might be for you?_____

_____

_____

_____

_____

OVERVIEW

The purpose of this chapter is to encourage helping professionals to see the overall benefits of supervision throughout the lifespan of the counseling career, value those benefits as a professional necessity, and eventually discover supervision approaches that fit their needs. The basic tenets and definitions of clinical counseling supervision will be presented, along with the roles, expectations, and functions of the supervisor/supervisee.

GOALS

- Understand the need for a holistic, integrative supervision book
- Define supervision and its major components
- Explain how clinical supervision is an integral part of professionalism

The Process of Supervision

The supervisor will usually clarify and combine three processes throughout supervision: roles, expectations, and functions. The roles that are used will be dependent on the supervisee's needs. During an informal or formal assessment, the supervisor may decide that the "hat" of the teacher, consultant, evaluator, and/or encourager is needed (Bernard & Goodyear, 1998).

Holloway and Carrol (1999) suggest that it is the supervision tasks and roles plus their functions that equal the supervision process. In other words, when the roles and responsibilities of the supervisor are combined with the need of the counselor in training, then a supervision process has begun.

During every supervision session the expectations must be clarified. Initially knowing what is expected from each member of the supervisory team is essential. The perceptions of the supervisor and supervisee will continue to be shared throughout the lifetime of supervisory experience. The functions of supervision will vary based upon the supervisee's needs as well. The major responsibilities, though, are that of administration, education, and support. A typical supervisory opening question might be, "What do you need and want out of supervision today?"(Russell-Chapin & Ivey, 2004).

Another essential mandate for a successful supervision experience is the proper documentation. In the appendices at the back of the book are examples of practicum/internship contracts, logs, consent forms and evaluations. Many institutions already use these types of forms.

The next category of forms is not often required. These newer forms will be included in the body of the chapter for further discussion. Whether the supervisee is a graduate student or a practicing counseling professional, some type of clinical supervision policy and supervision plan is a must. Both the written supervision policy and the supervision plan assist in clarifying the expectations, tasks, and roles in the supervision relationship. The two examples below are ones the authors use in their private practice.

Resource Management Services, Inc.

CLINICAL SUPERVISION POLICY
(Draft)

1. All professional staff are required to participate in clinical supervision. Staff may choose from two supervision formats, individual or group. Group supervision will be provided twice a month (once a month in June, July, and August), at no cost to staff. Individual supervision must be arranged privately. All staff are required to attend group supervision a minimum of two hours a month or individual supervision one hour a month. Any other arrangement must be approved by the group's Chief Clinical Supervisor (CCS), Ted Chapin, PhD. Check your professional association's supervision requirement to determine how much supervision you need. Pressing clinical issues that cannot wait for scheduled supervision are to be brought to immediate supervisory attention.

2. All supervisory discussions will be appropriately documented and filed with the CCS. The documentation is to include the date, counselor name, client name, supervisory issue, recommended action, and, as indicated, resolution. In addition, the name of each person attending supervision will also be noted.

3. All clinical staff are expected to follow their respective professional ethical guidelines and are further required to give special attention to the following primary clinical duties, presenting any such issue for immediate supervision.

   a. Duty to prevent client from harming self or others
   b. Duty to protect client confidentiality

    c. Duty to provide for client continuity of service

    d. Duty to keep adequate clinical records

    e. Duty to properly diagnose and treat clients

    f. Duty to avoid dual relationships and sexual impropriety

    All office staff (clerical, accounting, data management, and administrative) must also, as appropriate, follow and/or be mindful of the above primary duties, presenting any such issue to their immediate supervisor for feedback, clarification, and/or appropriate action.

4. All clinical staff are to make reasonable arrangements for their client's care should they be unavailable due to vacation or illness. This includes notification to the on-call person of clients who may be in crisis while they are not available and notice to clients who are in crisis that they will not be available, but an on-call staff will be available to help them. Any resulting incidents are to be appropriately documented and forwarded to the primary therapist at earliest possible notice.

5. All clinical staff are required to complete a professional will that outlines the actions to be taken for the care of their clients and their records, and compensation due should they become functionally incapacitated or deceased (see attached example).

6. All staff are covered for any professional acts of malpractice by the organization's liability insurance policy. This does not limit individual staff from maintaining their own liability policies at their own expense. Should any staff receive notice of a licensing board complaint or a potential legal action being filed, they should immediately apprise the CCS.

7. Finally, it is also understood that the clinical supervisor's role may include, as necessary, the audit of staff client records, review of staff client satisfaction surveys, assessment of staff clinical competency, and investigation of complaints brought forward against an individual staff person. It is further understood that the primary intent of any oversight action will be to assess the situation, discuss the matter with the given staff person, and resolve the presenting clinical problem.

    Should the problem involve a more serious ethical infraction, the clinical supervisor may also require remedial action including but not limited to continuing education, individual supervision, restriction or limitation of professional duties, reporting to the respective staff person's licensing board, and/or termination of employment. Staff may appeal any remedial requirement by submitting such a request in writing to the CCS. A panel of three colleagues, selected by the CCS, will review the appeal.

It is understood that the goal of the RMS Clinical Supervision Policy is to guard the quality and care of client treatment by supporting, monitoring, and correcting any action that could be harmful to a client, jeopardize a staff person's professional standing, impede a supervisor's role, effect the group's reputation and standing in the community, and/or present a risk of liability to individual staff members, clinical supervisors, or the group practice. In this spirit, your signature below indicates your understanding, commitment to, and compliance with the guidelines and requirements noted above.

_____　　_____　　_____　　_____

Staff Signature　　　　　　　　*Date*　　　　　*Chief Clinical Supervisor*　　　*Date*

If the supervisee is a graduate student, some type of Internship Supervision Contract must be utilized. The forms in the appendices of this book are examples from a packet of information each intern is given in the graduate program at Bradley University. All of these forms provide structure and guidance for successfully engaging the supervisory process. See Appendix A.

The Supervision Plan

The supervisee and supervisor can develop two plans, if needed. The first is a long-range plan spelling out long-term goals. The second supervision plan creates a format for individual supervision sessions. The formats can also be personally developed, but the following need to be included in the plans: supervision goals and question for each session, outcomes, developmental needs of the client and supervisee, multicultural issues, diagnosis/conceptualization, evaluations, and supervision notes (Stoltenberg & Pace, 2008; Russell-Chapin, 2007).

Discussion Questions 2

1. At this moment, what do you want out of your clinical supervision? Be sure to complete the Supervision Policy and Plan with your supervisor. _____

   _____

   _____

   _____

   _____

2. What expectations need to be clarified to make the supervisory experience successful?

   _____

   _____

   _____

   _____

Supervision Foundational Elements

Ellis (2006) conducted a research study using naturalistic data to examine the Loganbill, Hardy, and Delworth (1982) and the Sansbury (1982) hierarchical models and found that supervisory relationship, competence, emotional awareness, and autonomy are essential variable for training supervisors. The authors concur with Ellis and additionally structure their supervision with six essential foundational elements that most supervision sessions must address: expectations, multicultural differences between the supervisor and supervisee, supervisory questions, selection of supervision approach dependent upon supervision question, multiaxial diagnosis and conceptualization/interventions, and supervisory outcomes. Therefore, these elements will be addressed and demonstrated throughout the text and DVD examples:

1. Clarify supervision expectations and building supervisory relationships
2. Explore multicultural backgrounds; similarities and differences
3. Listen to supervisory questions
4. Select an appropriate supervision approach
5. Discuss diagnosis/conceptualization
6. Analyze supervisory outcomes

Categories of Supervision

The two major categories of supervision are clinical and administrative. Although the functions of the categories often overlap, the focus of each is distinct. Clinical supervision emphasizes the services, direct and indirect, that a supervisee provides to clients. Clinical supervision usually means face-to-face supervision promoting supervisee development, working on counseling skills in the counseling relationship, advocating for the client's best interest, conceptualization, diagnosis, and prognosis (Powell, 1993).

Administrative supervision has its focus on the roles and responsibilities that the supervisee must provide to the organization, agency, or employer (Tromski-Klingshirn & Davis, 2007; Bradley & Kottler, 2001). Tromski-Klingshirn (2006) states that there are many role conflicts and role ambiguity issues when the same person is the clinical supervisor and the administrative supervisor. However, in recent research by Tromski-Klingshirn (2007) 70 counselor supervisees who were working on the second tier of their state licensure responded to a study about dual supervisory roles. Forty-nine percent reported that their main clinical supervisor was also their administrative supervisor; 51 percent stated that the primary clinical supervisor was not the administrative supervisor. After the data were analyzed, no statistical group differences were found. Generally, what supervisees thought about the dual roles tended to hover around the attributes and attitudes of the individuals involved in supervision more than their roles.

In the world of the counselor, this administrative aspect might have to be handled by the same person, for the smooth functioning of the organization. It is the authors' opinion that, if possible, clinical supervision is still best achieved from a supervisor who does not have administrative and/or evaluative functions. The supervisee can then focus on honest fears and insecurities, without concern about job performance, merit raises, and reprisals. Perhaps the best solution is a combination of supervision from within and outside of the organization.

Supervision and Professionalism

All of the helping professions use some type of clinical supervision to assist students and helping professionals alike in developing new counseling skills, maintaining current skills, and building professional competencies (Haynes, Corey, & Moulton, 2003). The use of clinical supervision seems universal, but the manner in which professionals conduct supervision varies widely.

The counseling profession, like any discipline offering a public service, has a responsibility to assess continually the quality of the service. It is also the responsibility of the counselor to analyze the degree to which counseling is helping clients and its overall effectiveness and outcome (Nugent, 1990). As Neukrug (2003) so eloquently stated, "Embracing a professional lifestyle does not end once one finishes graduate school, obtains a job, becomes licensed, has 10 years of experience or becomes a 'master therapist.' It is a lifelong commitment to a way of being, a way that says you are constantly striving to make yourself a better person and a more effective counselor, committed to professional activities" (p. 72).

Supervision over the Lifespan of a Counseling Career

Any supervisor and supervisee must have the supervision theory and skills to adjust to the needs of clients. For many years in the supervision world, that has not been the case. There has been a long-standing idea that good counselors make good supervisors. If the counselors understand the world of counseling, then they will understand the world of supervision. There are many problems with that assumption (Gazzola & Theriault, 2007). One problem is that relying on the counseling process to facilitate the supervision process may not be appropriate and could lead to damaging supervisory experiences (Ladany, 2004). Historically, few supervisors have been trained in supervision. Without proper supervision training, many helping professionals often become comfortable and perhaps complacent and even safe in the views of how counseling and supervision should be accomplished.

The current view of supervision is that clinical supervision is emerging as a separate field of knowledge with a distinct skill set of theories, skills, and processes (Bernard & Goodyear, 2007). Another recent change is that one of the most exciting and fruitful methods of achieving the goal of becoming a seasoned helping professional is to engage in clinical supervision throughout the lifespan of a counseling career (Grant & Schofield, 2007). For many counselors, clinical supervision began in graduate school, and once the program of study was completed, so were the days of supervision (Russell-Chapin, 2007). The material in this book will hopefully convince and encourage students, faculty, and helping professionals to understand the benefits of incorporating supervision across the lifespan of our counseling careers, whether that career is as a supervisor, supervisee, or both.

Although there is a paucity of research studies that focus on supervision throughout the counseling career, Townend, Ianetta, and Freeston (2002) conducted a survey of 280 randomly selected members of the British Association of Behavioural and Cognitive Psychotherapists. Ninety percent of the sample met the supervision requirements of the association and were very satisfied with their supervisory experience. In England, 72 percent of the 127 psychologists surveyed received post-qualification supervision, but only 18 percent were satisfied with the supervisory arrangements (Gabbay, 1999).

Discussion Questions 3

1. What are the benefits that you see from continuing supervision over the life span of a counseling career?_____

_____

_____

_____

_____

2. What might the disadvantages be if supervision were not continued?_____

_____

_____

_____

_____

Supervision Advocacy

Supervision advocacy is now in the spotlight because many see the benefits of supervision over the life span of a career. Lori found this to be true in returning to supervision on her university sabbatical. Ted has always continued in supervision since he began practicing over 25 years ago. Supervision continues to refresh, rejuvenate, and keep us on the cutting edge. If more helping professions will view supervision as an ongoing cutting-edge practice, then the counseling profession will also become more accountable and outcome effective (Russell-Chapin, 2007).

The concept of supervision has changed over the years. Although supervision of counseling interns has always been a constant, now many helping professions are requiring supervision courses in their curricula, and many state licensing boards are mandating that all renewing and newly licensed professionals have additional coursework in supervision.

As more helping professions understand the benefits of supervision over the life span of a counseling career, graduate curricula and state statutes governing licensure will continue to change and grow. In the state of Illinois, renewal of licensure now depends upon earning 18 contact hours of supervision training. When asked the reason behind this new requirement, the board stated that most of the grievances came about because of poor or inadequate supervision. Because Lori has been conducting supervision workshops throughout the state and nation, she began collecting ideas from all the supervision experts and participants encountered. One of the first interactive group questions asked was "What are the best and worst traits of the supervisors you have encountered?"

In Table 1.1, readers can see the cumulative answers to this question. The following qualities seemed to be the main responses from approximately 500 supervisors and supervisees:

TABLE 1.1　Best and Worst Traits of Supervisors

Best Supervisor Experience	Worst Supervisor Experience
Available	Blaming
Beside you (mentor)	Condescending
Calm and warm	Controlling
Caring	Critical
Challenging	Defensive
Collaborative	Distracted
Comfortable and positive	Distracting
Providing constructive feedback	Inspiring fear
Creative	Impaired
Enabling developmental awareness	Having inadequate skills
Empathetic	Making inappropriate jokes
Encouraging	Insensitive
Equal	Lacking advice
Promoting equal power	Lacking balance
Fun	Manipulative
Humble and wise	Making one feel micromanaged
Humorous	Mismatched
Nonjudgmental	Narrow-minded
Presenting options	Being unavailable
Protecting the profession	Not giving feedback
Reciprocal	Not listening
Resourceful	Not providing options
Respectful	Nonengaging
"Saw the best in me"	Inflexible
Secure	Not validating
Sharing ideas	Political
Having a solid knowledge base	Snapping fingers
Strategic	Using stereotypes
Giving suggestions	Too much trouble
Supportive	Too opinionated
Inspiring trust	Unethical
Validating	Unwelcoming

Introduction to DVD Demonstrations

Please access the first segments of the DVD. The first DVD segment is titled Introduction as it is the history behind all the demonstrations. Below is the actual transcript of the introduction.

Hi, My name is Dr. Lori Russell-Chapin, and I have been teaching and supervising graduate students at Bradley University in Peoria, Illinois, for the past 19 years. Last year I was on sabbatical, and I decided to return to a supervision group as a supervisee. What I discovered was that I enjoy being a supervisee as much as I love being a supervisor.

The concept of supervision has changed over the years. Now many helping professions are requiring supervision courses in their curricula, and many state licensing boards are mandating that all licensed professionals have additional coursework in supervision. This new thought arose out of several grievance procedures where poor supervision was being received.

Supervision advocacy is also in the forefront because many see the benefits of supervision over the life span of a career. I found this to be true in returning to supervision. Supervision continues to refresh, rejuvenate, and keep me on the cutting edge. If more helping professions will view supervision as an ongoing must, then the counseling profession will also become more accountable and outcome effective.

Today the viewers will hear five individual case studies with five unique helping professionals who are at different points in their careers. Each case and counselor have differing needs and demands, so I will demonstrate five separate models of supervision that are relevant to the supervision needs. The definition I am using for supervision is it is a distinct approach and response to supervisees' needs from a supervisor who often has more technical expertise and wisdom. The main goal is for viewers to understand that many unique supervision methods and models exist that correspond to basic supervisee needs. Perhaps there is a model that could be helpful to each of you.

Summary

This chapter focused on the manner in which you can use this textbook, a working definition of supervision, and the impact of supervision over the life span of a helping professional career. Readers need to understand that many unique supervision methods and models exist that correspond to basic supervisee needs. A major goal of this textbook is to assist helping professionals in expanding their knowledge base for supervision and discovering models of supervision that can allow them to respond more effectively and flexibly, whether the role is of supervisor and/or supervisee. This first chapter also offers several forms to assist in providing structure, expectations, and roles.

Chapter One Final Discussion Questions

1. Please answer the following question. Think back to your best and worst supervisory experiences in any work/life experience. What were the qualities of the best supervisors and worst supervisors? If your answers are not in the Chapter One table, be sure to write to Lori and Ted, so we can add your comments to the list. _____

_____

_____

_____

2. As you write down your best supervisor qualities, a profile of a healthy supervisor begins to emerge. Are these the same supervisory traits that you see yourself exhibiting? Explore. _____

_____

_____

_____

References

Bernard, J. M., & Goodyear, R. K. (1998). *Fundamentals of clinical supervision.* Needham Heights, MA: Allyn and Bacon.

Bernard, J. M., & Goodyear, R. K. (2004). *Fundamentals of clinical supervision,* 3rd ed. Boston: Allyn & Bacon.

Bernard, J. M., & Goodyear, R. K. (2008). *Fundamentals of clinical supervision,* 4th ed. Needham Heights, MA: Allyn & Bacon.

Bradley, L. J., & Kottler, J. A. (2001). *Overview of counselor supervision.* In L. J. Bradley and N. Ladany (Eds.), *Counselor supervision: Principles, process and practice* (3rd ed.). Philadelphia: Brunner-Routledge.

Ellis, M. V. (2006). Critical incidents in clinical supervision and in supervisor supervision: Assessing supervisory issues, *Training and Education in Professional Psychology,* v. S(2), 122–132.

Gabbay, M. B., Kiemle, G., & Maguire, C. (1999). Clinical supervision for clinical psychologists: Existing provision and unmet needs. *Clinical Psychology and Psychotherapy,* 6, 404–412.

Gazzola, N., & Theriault, A. (2007). Relational themes in counselling supervision: Broadening and narrowing processes, *Canadian Journal of Counselling.* 41, 228–243.

Grant, J., & Schofield, M. (2007). Career-long supervision: Patterns and perspectives. *Counselling and Psychotherapy,* 7, 3–11, British Association for Counselling and Psychotherapy.

Haynes, R., Corey, G., & Moulton, P. (2003). *Clinical supervision in the helping professions: A practical guide.* Pacific Grove, CA: Brooks/Cole.

Holloway, E., & Carrol, M. (Eds.) (1999). *Training clinical supervisors: Strategies, methods and techniques.* London, England: Sage Publications.

Ladany, N. (2004). Psychotherapy supervision: What lies beneath. *Psychotherapy Research,* 14, 1–19.

Loganbill, C., Hardy, E., & Delworth, U. (1982). Supervision: A conceptual model. *The Counseling Psychologist, 10,* 3–42.

Neukrug, E. (2003). *The world of the counselor.* Pacific Grove, CA: Brooks/Cole-Thomson Learning.

Nugent, F. (1990). *An introduction to the profession of counseling.* Columbus, OH: Merrill Publishing.

Powell, D. J. (1993). *Clinical supervision in alcohol and drug abuse counseling: Principles, models, methods.* New York: Lexington Books.

Russell-Chapin, L. A. (2007). Supervision: An essential for professional counselor development. In J. Gregoire & C. M. Jungers (Eds.), *The counselor's companion: What every beginning counselor needs to know* (pp. 79–80). Mahwah, NJ: Lawrence Erlbaum.

Russell-Chapin, L. A., & Ivey, A. E. (2004). *Your supervised practicum and internship: Field resources for turning theory into action.* Pacific Grove, CA: Brooks/Cole.

Sansbury, D. L. Developmental supervision from a skills perspective. (1982). *The Counseling Psychologist 10, 1,* 53–57.

Stoltenberg, C. D., & Pace, T. M. (2008). Science and practice in supervision: An evidence-based practice in psychology approach in W. B. Walsh (Ed.). *Biennial Review of Counseling Psychology.* American Psychological Association, Society of Counseling Psychology, Division 17. New York: Psychology Press.

Townend, M., Iannetta, K., & Freeston, M. H. (2002). Clinical supervision in practice: A survey of UK cognitive behavioural psychotherapists accredited by the BABCP. *Behavioural and Cognitive Psychotherapy, 30,* 485–500.

Tromski-Klingshirn, D. (2006). Should the clinical supervisor be the administrative supervisor? *The Clinical Supervisor, 25,* 53–67.

Tromski-Klingshirn, D. M., & Davis, T. E. (2007). Supervisee's perceptions of their clinical supervision: A study of the dual role of clinical and administrative supervisor. *Counselor Education and Supervision, 46,* 294–304.

Obstacles to Effective Supervision

Supervisee Factors

Preparation

Supervisees enter supervision from a variety of levels of preparation, and each brings their own opportunities and potential obstacles. Some supervisees are students, who typically have little experience, much excitement, some idealism and lots of anxiety. In the middle of the spectrum are new or junior professionals; they have some experience and are likely looking to fulfill qualifications for licensure or certification. They often bring more preconceptions about therapy and supervision, and their expectations are often more well formed than students'. At the far end of the spectrum are experienced, senior professionals, who very frequently have a clear idea of what they want out of supervision. They may be more focused and thus closed-minded about the range of possible benefits supervision can provide.

On a more behavioral level, a very real obstacle to supervision is a supervisee's lack of preparation for the supervision session. Did the supervisee take time to review her caseload, select a case for review, write up a thorough case summary report, decide where she was struggling and conclude what they wanted supervision to address? Ironically, students, although less experienced, are often more disciplined in preparing for supervision than their more experienced counterparts. Their academic programs have likely demanded that they organize their work, and this has created a more disciplined approach to preparation. More experienced, employed professionals are fitting supervision into their busy schedules. They may have a very focused agenda for supervision such as a particular client they are struggling with concerning a question about diagnosis, intervention ideas, or medication issues. Lack of more thorough preparation will likely limit the supervisor's ability to offer a sound response. It is one of the supervisor's responsibilities to formulate, early on in supervision, a mutually agreed upon set of supervisory guidelines and expectation.

Confidence

While student supervisees are learning and acquiring their professional confidence, they can become hindered by their reluctance to take appropriate risks. For example, perhaps they suspect a client may be suicidal but are afraid to ask, so they don't. In supervision the issue comes up, and the supervisee hides his avoidance from the supervisor. The opportunity for deeper learning may be missed. With more experienced supervisees, lack of confidence or unwillingness to take appropriate risks may cause them to avoid developing new skills or trying a new intervention technique. Effective supervision for more experienced professionals is not only about fulfilling credentialing or licensing requirements or maintaining the status quo, it's also about continued growth and professional development. The supervisory relationship provides an ideal environment for learning, application, and feedback. If professional counselors cannot stretch their skills there, where can they?

OVERVIEW

Effective supervision can be viewed as an optimal combination of four important factors. These factors include the supervisee, supervisor, the supervisory relationship, and the structural elements of supervision. The supervisee brings with them a set of personal and professional needs as well a capacity or readiness to benefit from the supervisory experience. The supervisor brings a set of abilities, skills, experience, and knowledge that prepares them to function as an effective mentor. The supervisory relationship involves the quality of match between the supervisee and supervisor. It is initially formed through careful pre-supervision selection and screening and is enhanced by the creation of a healthy supervisory chemistry. This relationship factor is one of the few elements that all supervision models agree upon (Holloway, 1995; Morgan & Sprenkle, 2007). Although perhaps more subtle, the structural aspects of the supervision setting, such as available equipment, facility constraints, and professional staff support are also important. The purpose of this chapter is to explore each of these factors, the potential obstacles they present for effective supervision, and some suggestions on how these obstacles can either be avoided or appropriately managed should they arise. The reader may find that some of the following issues will bring to mind other potential obstacles that are not fully addressed in this chapter. Should that occur, the principles outlined here may provide a helpful guide for how these too can be successfully resolved.

GOALS

- Identify potential obstacles toward effective supervision

- Offer resources to counteract obstacles

Defensiveness

The word, supervision, in our culture has become synonymous with evaluation; evaluation can be intimidating (Russell-Chapin & Ivey, 2004). There is an obvious level of vulnerability present in the supervisory relationship, especially when a student supervisee works with an experienced senior clinician. This vulnerability, however, is also present when a senior professional works with a supervisor she considers her colleague. "If I disclose my flaws or short-comings to this colleague, what will he think of me?" Sometimes, even asking a question can become an admission of doubt or a notice of something lacking. Defensiveness can become a serious obstacle to effective supervision.

Underlying defensiveness is insecurity and mistrust. Although most supervisees will bring to supervision their personal level of security or insecurity, mistrust will become magnified if the supervisory relationship becomes a place of humiliation or judgment. It is very important for supervision to be a safe place to explore self-doubt, take appropriate risks, be open to feedback, and learn from our experiences. This requires the supervisee to trust, self-disclose, listen, and react nondefensively to feedback. It also requires the supervisor to be empathetic, reassuring, and encouraging. This does not mean avoiding the difficult conversations, but rather handling them in an honest, direct, genuine, and caring manner. This will allow the supervisee to comfortably face his insecurity and the supervisor to fulfill her obligation toward the competent practice of the profession.

Another method for decreasing the power differential between the supervisee and supervisor is to offer the supervisee the opportunity to openly discuss the supervisory experience and to evaluate the supervisor. Usually evaluation tends to be one-sided. The supervisee understands that she will be evaluated, but Downs (2000) suggests providing continuous evaluations of the supervisor may heighten the supervisee's investment in the supervision process and decrease anxiety.

Unresolved Personal Issues

One of the most difficult but most important and powerful issues to face in supervision is when unresolved personal supervisee issues make themselves obvious in a counseling relationship. Some of these include therapists with anxious attachment styles (Beutler, Blatt, Alimohamed, Levi, & Angtuaco, 2006) and personal hostility (Henry, Strupp, Butler, Schact, & Binder, 1993) that may impede therapeutic empathy, as well as other therapist vulnerabilities, including excessive need to be liked or admired and inability to receive criticism (Wolberg, 1967); difficulty tolerating negative emotion (Strupp & Hadley, 1985); and difficulty admitting and correcting errors committed during treatment (Greenson, 1967).

It takes courage for the supervisor to address issues, and it takes humility for the supervisee to acknowledge it. Left unaddressed, it can become the "pink elephant in the living room" that everyone sees but dares not talk about. Ethically we understand our limits in being able to help a client when we ourselves are struggling, perhaps unsuccessfully, with the same issue. We are hand-tied by our blind spots, biased in our positions, and often limited in our ability to consider an alternate response. Unresolved personal issues should become resolved personal issues and frequently require the supervisee to get counseling and to limit her work with this type of problem until she is better able to be effective. If the supervisee is impaired and could do or has done harm to clients, then appropriate action must take place. Rapisarda and Britton (2007) conducted a qualitative study regarding the efficacy of sanctioned supervision for the impaired counselor. The results of their focus groups show promise for the effectiveness of sanctioned supervision, if the necessary training for supervisors is provided. The authors of this study state, "The counseling profession has recognized the importance of identifying and intervening when counselors may be providing sub-standard care to clients" (p. 82). Counseling professional organizations support the intervention of counselor impairment through their ethical guidelines by stipulating that best practices and best interest of clients is the goal (American Counseling Association, 2005; American Mental Health Association, 2010; American Psychological Association, 2002; and National Association of Social Workers, 1999).

Several of the recommendations to help impaired helping professionals are advocating for lifelong supervision, encouraging supervisors to be gatekeepers of the counseling profession, emphasizing the importance of wellness and stress reduction, supporting supervisors who take action on subquality counseling, and increasing evaluation and research efforts in the area of counselor impairment (Russell-Chapin, 2007; Cobia & Pipes, 2002; Thomas, 2005).

The supervisory role in the case of impairment is to be supportive yet firm. The supervisor must set the boundaries regarding appropriate behavior and the supervisee must be willing to get help with his unresolved personal issues. This is not a problem to be met with shame or self-doubt but rather with responsible action that will strengthen the supervisee personally and professionally enhance her competency.

Discussion Question 1

Of the supervisee factors listed above, which one(s) may be your biggest obstacle toward effective supervision? _____

_____

_____

_____

_____

Supervisor Factors

Competency

The first and perhaps most critical supervisor factor is the supervisor's training and competence in providing effective supervision. There are many ways that a supervisor can develop his competence. Supervisors can take formal graduate coursework in clinical supervision from an accredited institution. This will typically expose them to supervision theory and practice. Supervisors can also receive supervision of their supervision from an experienced and qualified colleague who has established credentials in provided supervision of supervision. Another path to competency involves the attendance of professional workshops or seminars on clinical supervision. Many states now require 18 or more contact hours in supervision continuing education for renewal of state licenses. Finally, the Center for Credentialing and Education (CCE, 2001) offers an Approved Clinical Supervision (ACS) certification. This involves completion of an application, a processing fee, and submission and review of an audio/video case presentation with multiaxial diagnosis.

Nonspecific Feedback

Supervision between colleagues is a very useful and often convenient means of clinical supervision. However, in some situations, strong mutual interests in maintaining a respectful and friendly professional relationship can mute effective collegial supervision. This bind can potentially place the friendship above focused supervision and result in feedback that may be too general or vague and not specific enough to be of any meaningful help to the supervisee. It is important that supervisors feel free and able to give the quality and depth of feedback that will help the supervisee improve her skills.

Narrow Scope of Supervision

Some supervisors have a narrowly defined definition of supervision that significantly limits the supervisory opportunity for the supervisee. Sometimes supervision is limited to case conceptualization, diagnosis, and treatment planning. Although useful, this does not address the myriad of issues that could be explored in supervision. Some of these include enhancement of micro skills, the therapeutic relationship, theoretically based insights, self in the counseling process, transference and counter-transference issues, projection, alternative interventions, potentially harmful effects of treatment, ethics, and referral options. It is up to the supervisor to manage the supervision session in such a way that there is an opportunity to address each of the above issues. By expanding the scope of supervision, the supervisee will be more fully trained and prepared to offer effective clinical services to his clients.

In order to expand the scope of supervision, however, the culture and expectations of supervision must also expand. Supervision must assist in clinical competency and growth and help the profession and consumer to understand that the counseling profession takes serious steps for monitoring and preserving quality (Crocket, 2007; Falender & Shafranske, 2004; Feltham, 2000). Expanding the scope of supervision seems to be a European concern as well (West & Clark, 2004; Besley & Edwards, 2005).

Excessive Criticism

When a supervisee enters each supervision session, he is taking a risk in exposing his clinical limitations and, sometimes, relevant personal issues. If a supervisor is too harsh, too confrontative, or too punitive in her style of feedback, the supervisee will likely feel threatened and withdraw. The challenge for the supervisor is to be direct, focused, and encouraging. Although the content of supervision must be addressed, the supervisory relationship also requires proper attention or the entire process will break down.

Discussion Question 2

Of the supervisor factors listed, which one(s) will be the most important for you as the supervisor and supervisee? _____

_____

_____

_____

_____

Supervisory Relationship

Personality Conflicts

Although great effort is usually exercised in the formation of a good supervisory relationship, sometimes differences in personality undermine the essential development of rapport between a supervisor and supervisee. If attempts to overcome these differences fail, the supervisory relationship is bound to suffer and little effective supervision can be done (Fall & Sutton, 2004). Although personality conflicts can disrupt the supervisory process, they can also present an opportunity for great learning and growth. By working through these differences, the supervisee and supervisor will likely be more effective in working with their own diverse client base. As therapists, we do not always like every client who comes through the door, but we must learn how to work with them or we will severely limit our practice. However, as in therapy, should we find that the personality conflicts we encounter in clinical supervision cannot be successfully resolved and will continue to diminish the quality of supervision, we must end this supervisory relationship and find another with a more complimentary blend of personalities.

Mismatch of Theoretical Orientations

The theoretical orientations of professional counselors vary by training, supervision, and personal preference. Many theoretical orientations are anchored in time and through historical popularity. For example, a Rogerian-oriented therapist may have been trained in the 1960s, whereas a strategic therapist may have been trained in the 1990s. Both bring a very distinct set of assumptions about the process and mechanisms of change, some of which are likely at sharp odds with one another. A mismatch of theoretical orientations could be both an opportunity for learning from each other's style and a source of much frustration and potential conflict should either the supervisor or supervisee stubbornly hold fast to his or her own theoretical world view. As with other issues in clinical supervision, differences of theoretical orientation are best addressed before the supervisory relationship is established. This allows for clarification of expectations and an informed decision before entering into the supervision contract.

As noted above, there can be a great opportunity for learning through differing theoretical orientations. The various perspectives, underlying assumptions, and related intervention strategies may well expand and enrich a supervisee's background and skill set. Still, if a supervisee is looking to gain more depth in a particular theoretical orientation, then the match between supervisor and supervisee becomes most important, and depth of learning will be assured.

Diversity Issues

As in the practice of psychotherapy, diversity issues also present a potential obstacle in the supervisory relationship. Differences in culture, ethnicity, religion, age, gender, and sexual orientation could undermine the relationship if not properly understood and integrated into the supervisory relationship. Diversity issues affect values, perspective, behavior, and communication styles. It is vitally important for the supervisor to have some training in diversity and how to handle these issues in supervision. It is also important for the supervisee to understand how diversity may affect the relationship with his or her supervisor. One way of enhancing one's skill in handling diversity is to seek out continuing education on counseling and supervision with diverse populations. Another is to be prepared to engage a process of active discovery in learning and understanding these differences through the suspension of assumptions and open communication about differences. Diversity can be a rich source of understanding for both the supervisor and supervisee.

The emphasis on multicultural/diversity training in counseling programs has heightened our awareness and skill levels. It is commonplace for supervisees and supervisors to be better informed about personal biases and prejudices (Doughty & Leddick, 2007). However, gender bias of supervisees and supervisors is often overlooked. Chung, Marshall, and Gordon (2001) strongly recommend that gender bias must also be addressed with supervisees and supervisors. In their study, they found that male supervisors were more likely to give a negative evaluation for female supervisees than males. Granello (2003) discovered that supervisors of both genders requested male supervisee's thoughts and opinions two times more than they did with a female counterpart. The flip side was that when female supervisees offered suggestions, both male and female supervisors were more likely to use those suggestions to create a new idea than with male supervisees.

Once again it is essential to the supervisory relationship that issues of diversity be addressed in the beginning of the relationship. Gatmon, Jackson, Koshkarian, and Marty-Perry (2001) conducted a study of 289 predoctoral psychology interns and discovered that supervisees who discussed gender issues such as similarities and differences were overall more satisfied with the quality of their supervision.

Inattention to Potentially Harmful Effects of Treatment

Although it is recognized that there is established research evidence that psychotherapy works, it is less recognized that there is also evidence that some clients fail to benefit and others even deteriorate while in treatment (Lambert & Ogles, 2004). Lilienfeld (2007) called for renewed attention to the potentially deleterious effects of psychotherapy as a crucial aspect of effective practice. Castonguay, Boswell, Constantino, Goldfried, and Hill (2010) detailed a working list of some 20 recommendations for minimizing these potentially harmful effects. These recommendations fell into five categories, including enhancing the therapeutic relationship, appropriate use of empirically supported treatments and techniques, prevention and repair of toxic therapy relationships and technical processes, the adjustment of treatment choice and outcome expectations due to client characteristics and type of problem, and therapist treatment for unresolved personal problems that impede his or her effectiveness.

It is of course vital that the supervisory relationship be strong enough to address these issues. Both supervisees and supervisors need to be aware of the potentially harmful effects of psychotherapy treatment and be ready to implement strategies for avoiding or minimizing possible harm to clients.

Failure to Utilize Outcome Data

The failure to utilize objective therapy outcome and process feedback can significantly reduce therapeutic and supervisory effectiveness. These valuable tools help assess signs of improvement or decline. Lambert (2007) found simple, session-by-session feedback can help identify and decrease rates of therapeutic deterioration. There are a number of instruments designed to do this, two of which are the Outcome Questionnaire (Lambert, 2007) and the Treatment Outcome Package (Kraus, Seligman, & Jordan, 2005). The most effective instruments should be brief, user friendly, and acceptable to clients, supervisees, and supervisors.

Other instruments have been designed to assess the quality of the therapeutic relationship, therapist's level of engagement, client's openness to the experience, and critical incidents in therapy (Greenberg & Pinsof, 1986; Hill & Lambert, 2004; and Llewelyn, 1988). Effective supervision includes an assessment of client progress. This allows supervisees to become aware of their ongoing impact on clients, to better understand their strengths and weaknesses, and to alter their therapeutic approach. Objective outcome and process feedback thus improves supervisee skill and therapeutic results.

Lack of Ethics

Unethical behavior can destroy a supervisory relationship as quickly as it does a therapeutic relationship. It is the supervisors' responsibility to understand and apply the ethical guidelines for the provision of supervision as defined by their respective professional associations. It is also important for the supervisee to be informed of the ethical guidelines of clinical supervision so as to be both knowledgeable and confident about their use in supervision. Should an infraction become evident, it is necessary to provide specific feedback to the offending party, outline the ethical guideline, and request future compliance. Should these efforts fail, the recourse is to file a complaint with the offending party's professional association, credentialing board, and/or state licensing agency. Ethics are meant to protect clients, supervisees, and the integrity of the profession. There is no room for unethical behavior in the supervisory relationship. However, as the supervision scope grows, the counseling profession must also recognize the challenging legal and ethical consequences of supervisory demands and expectations. (Cobia & Boes, 2000).

Formality

An overly formal supervisory style can seriously inhibit the supervisory relationship and limit supervisee clinical education. Many times, a more experienced and senior professional colleague will provide supervision. This colleague will likely have status over the supervisee. This colleague may be a college professor, an employer, or a clinical director. For effective supervision to occur, these professional boundaries and the formality they often engender should be set aside to allow space for rapport, trust, and essential interpersonal aspects of the supervisory relationship to develop. Supervisees will likely remember the encouragement, personal support, and confidence their supervisor helped instill in them, rather than the status of supervisor's position or even their expert insights into a particular case. As in psychotherapy, being human, genuine, and self-disclosing provides the supervisee a safe place to learn, fail, and become an even more skilled therapist.

Discussion Questions 3

1. As outlined in this section, there are many factors influencing the supervisory relationship. Which of these will be the most difficult to discuss in this relationship?

_____

_____

_____

_____

_____

2. Discuss the importance of emphasizing the differing diversity aspects in the supervisory relationship. _____

_____

_____

_____

_____

Structural Factors

Time

The commitment to supervision requires setting aside both scheduled meeting time and unscheduled consultation time. Most supervision is conducted within a typical therapy hour format.

Group supervision may be scheduled up to 1½ hours in length. Unscheduled consultation time may involve telephone calls, e-mails, or quick drop-in visits. Time can become an obstacle if the supervisor is tightly scheduled, runs late for appointments, or is unavailable outside of scheduled appointments. As with any professional obligation, it is important for the supervisor to make sure he can fulfill the needs of the supervisee or the supervisee may become frustrated, and this could undermine the rapport between them. If a supervisor has agreed to supervise practicum or internship students, the supervisor must also expect to complete necessary paperwork issued by the student's academic program. The obligation to supervise another professional typically involves much more than an hour of supervision a week, so managing time is a very important supervisory skill.

Equipment

The classic supervision equipment primarily involved the use of a tape recorder. Today many training facilities use videotape, live observation through a two-way mirror with immediate "room to room" telephone communication, or remote viewing via a camera. These are the basic tools of supervision. Although most supervision involves conversation between the supervisor and supervisee, use of the above equipment can greatly improve the quality and depth of supervision. Audio tape, video recording, and live observation help to bring supervision into the "here and now." It is less likely that a supervisor will take the time to review a complete recording of a therapy session. Instead she will typically ask the supervisee to prepare in advance the parts of the recording the supervisee would like to discuss in supervision. This helps establish a focus for the supervision session and more accurately attends to the supervisee's needs. The lack of good supervision equipment can greatly hinder the supervisee's experience.

Setting

Clients seek psychotherapy in a variety of settings. Some of these include schools, colleges, health centers, hospitals, community mental health centers, private practices, hospices, and workplace settings. Each setting often directs its services to a particular type of clientele. These could include children, college students, medical patients, adults, chronically mentally ill, the dying, and employees. This range of practice setting and clientele offers many options to the supervisee seeking a particular kind of experience. Supervisors who have a similar interest and experience with a certain setting and clientele offer more focus to the supervisee. Each setting often has different norms of practice, unique environmental challenges, and sometimes a variety of allied professionals on its treatment team. Matching the supervisee and supervisor to the setting and clientele they prefer will improve supervision effectiveness. Mismatching will require a longer learning curve and potentially undermine the supervisee's experience.

Facility Support

As in any office setting, supervisees will need an appropriate facility from which to conduct their work. This means a private room, furniture, appropriate office supplies and forms, a telephone, and perhaps a computer. If a facility cannot provide these basic needs, then the supervisee is likely to feel like a second-class staff member and will struggle. Sometimes supervisees will share an office together or use whatever office is available. This can work, but the instability may increase anxiety and could fester into resentment. Supervisees are best treated as colleagues and provided all the necessary facility support they need, like any other professional staff member.

Staff Support

It is typically not enough for one member of a practice group to conduct clinical supervision without the support of the other group members. Everyone from the receptionist and office

TABLE 2.1   Supervisory Styles Inventory

For supervisee: Indicate your perception of the style of your current or most recent supervisor of psycho-therapy/counseling on each of the following descriptors. Circle the number on the scale, from 1 to 7, that best reflects your view of him or her.

For supervisors: Indicate your perceptions of your style as a supervisor of psychotherapy/counseling on each of the following descriptors. Circle the number on the scale, from 1 to 7, that best reflects your view of yourself.

	Supervisee							Supervisor						
	Not Very					Very		Not Very					Very	
1. Goal-oriented	1	2	3	4	5	6	7	1	2	3	4	5	6	7
2. Perceptive	1	2	3	4	5	6	7	1	2	3	4	5	6	7
3. Concrete	1	2	3	4	5	6	7	1	2	3	4	5	6	7
4. Explicit	1	2	3	4	5	6	7	1	2	3	4	5	6	7
5. Committed	1	2	3	4	5	6	7	1	2	3	4	5	6	7
6. Affirming	1	2	3	4	5	6	7	1	2	3	4	5	6	7
7. Practical	1	2	3	4	5	6	7	1	2	3	4	5	6	7
8. Sensitive	1	2	3	4	5	6	7	1	2	3	4	5	6	7
9. Collaborative	1	2	3	4	5	6	7	1	2	3	4	5	6	7
10. Intuitive	1	2	3	4	5	6	7	1	2	3	4	5	6	7
11. Reflective	1	2	3	4	5	6	7	1	2	3	4	5	6	7
12. Responsive	1	2	3	4	5	6	7	1	2	3	4	5	6	7
13. Structured	1	2	3	4	5	6	7	1	2	3	4	5	6	7
14. Evaluative	1	2	3	4	5	6	7	1	2	3	4	5	6	7
15. Friendly	1	2	3	4	5	6	7	1	2	3	4	5	6	7
16. Flexible	1	2	3	4	5	6	7	1	2	3	4	5	6	7
17. Prescriptive	1	2	3	4	5	6	7	1	2	3	4	5	6	7
18. Didactic	1	2	3	4	5	6	7	1	2	3	4	5	6	7
19. Thorough	1	2	3	4	5	6	7	1	2	3	4	5	6	7
20. Focused	1	2	3	4	5	6	7	1	2	3	4	5	6	7
21. Creative	1	2	3	4	5	6	7	1	2	3	4	5	6	7
22. Supportive	1	2	3	4	5	6	7	1	2	3	4	5	6	7
23. Open	1	2	3	4	5	6	7	1	2	3	4	5	6	7
24. Realistic	1	2	3	4	5	6	7	1	2	3	4	5	6	7
25. Resourceful	1	2	3	4	5	6	7	1	2	3	4	5	6	7
26. Invested	1	2	3	4	5	6	7	1	2	3	4	5	6	7
27. Facilitative	1	2	3	4	5	6	7	1	2	3	4	5	6	7
28. Therapeutic	1	2	3	4	5	6	7	1	2	3	4	5	6	7
29. Positive	1	2	3	4	5	6	7	1	2	3	4	5	6	7
30. Trusting	1	2	3	4	5	6	7	1	2	3	4	5	6	7
31. Informative	1	2	3	4	5	6	7	1	2	3	4	5	6	7
32. Humorous	1	2	3	4	5	6	7	1	2	3	4	5	6	7
33. Warm	1	2	3	4	5	6	7	1	2	3	4	5	6	7

Scoring key:
Attractive: Sum items 15, 16, 22, 23, 29, 30, 33; divide by 7.
Interpersonally sensitive: Sum items 2, 5, 10, 11, 21, 25, 26, 28; divide by 8.
Task oriented: Sum items 1, 3, 4, 7, 13, 14, 17, 18, 19, 20; divide by 10.
Filler items: 6, 8, 9, 12, 24, 27, 31, 32.

personnel to all of the clinical staff must be supportive. Supervisees will have many questions beyond the case material they bring for supervision. They may need to learn about schedul-ing, billing, access to computers, audiovisual equipment, office policies, release of information protocols, and community referral resources. They may also want to "pick the brains" of many professional staff, to learn about their areas of specialization. Support from the entire facility will be necessary for the supervisee to thrive. Although student supervisees, who are sure to make many mistakes, need the understanding and help of the whole staff, even professional supervisees will feel more supported if they are openly welcomed by the entire facility.

This chapter focuses on four main factors in supervision: the supervisor, the supervisee, the supervision relationship, and structural factors. Now that there is a better understanding of the factors of supervision, look over the inventory in Table 2.1, a Supervisory Styles Inventory (SSI) (Friedlander & Ward, 1984). Take the inventory as a supervisee and supervisor. Your results offer additional feedback to ensure there are fewer obstacles in the way of effective supervision.

As you score the results of the inventory, see whether your style fits the description from Friedlander and Ward (1984). Attractive supervisors are seen as warm, supportive, and often friendly. Interpersonally sensitive supervisors are seen as invested in the therapeutic process and what is happening to the supervisee. The task-oriented supervisor is seen as providing structure to the supervision session and focusing on goals and tasks (Russell-Chapin & Ivey, 2004).

According to Ladany, Marotta, and Muse-Burke (2001), as supervisees gain general experience, they become more adept at conceptualizing clients. In their research, the SSI was administered to supervisees measuring their perceptions of their supervisors. One of the outcomes of the research was that supervisees preferred supervisors who were moderately high on all three styles: attractive, interpersonally sensitive, and task oriented (Russell-Chapin & Ivey, 2004).

Discussion Questions 4

1. How are your responses different as a supervisor and a supervisee? _____

_____

_____

_____

2. These distinctions and similarities may be very important as you develop your own style. What have you discovered? _____

_____

_____

_____

Summary

The best way to ensure effective supervision is to take ample time to assess the match between the supervisor and supervisee upfront and to proactively attend to any mismatch issue that might derail the supervision. Supervisors should oversee all the necessary structural needs: managing time, supervision focus, facility and staff support. All supervisors should maintain a high level of competence and actively participate in continuing education to enhance their knowledge and skills. The supervisee should be ready, display a learning attitude, take responsibility for her part in the supervisory contract, be open to feedback, be assertive about her needs, and, when necessary, approach conflicts with the intention to resolve them. Finally, effective supervision is guaranteed when both the supervisor and supervisee are open to the wide array of personal and professional issues that find their way into a supervisory session. Few obstacles are impossible to overcome and can be readily managed with honesty, clear communication, a supportive and encouraging attitude, and a team approach.

Chapter Two Final Discussion Question

Which of the supervisory factors will provide the largest obstacle for you: the relationship or the structural elements? Write in depth about your concerns._____

_____

_____

_____

References

American Counseling Association. (2005). *ACA code of ethics and standards of practice.* Alexandria, VA: Author.

American Mental Health Counseling Association. (2010). *Code of ethics of the American Mental Health Counseling Association.* Alexandria, VA: Author.

American Psychological Association. (2002). *APA code of ethics and conduct.* Washington, DC: Author.

Besley, A.C. & Edwards, R. (2005). Editorial postsstructuralism and the impact of the work of Michel Foucalt in counselling and guidance. *British Journal of Guidance & Counselling, 33,* 277–281.

Beutler, L. E., Blatt, S. J., Alimohamed, S., Levy, K. N., & Angtuaco, L. (2006). Participant factors in treating dysphoric disorders. In L. G. Castonguay & L. E. Beutler (Eds.), *Principles of therapeutic change that work* (pp. 13–63). New York: Oxford University Press.

Castonguay, L. G., Boswell, J. F., Constantino, M. J., Goldfried, M. R., & Hill, C. E. (2010). Training implications of harmful effects of psychological treatments. *American Psychologist, 65,* 34–49.

Center for Credentialing and Education. (2001). Greensboro, NC: Author.

Chung, Y. B., Marshall, J. A., & Gordon, L. L. (2001). Racial and gender biases in supervisory evaluation and feedback. *The Clinical Supervisor, 20,* 99–111.

Cobia, D. C., & Boes, S. R. (2000). Professional disclosure statements and formal plans for supervision: Two strategies for minimizing the risk of ethical conflicts in postmaster's supervision. *Journal of Counseling and Development, 78,* 293–296.

Cobia, D. C., & Pipes, R. B. (2002). Mandated supervision: An intervention for disciplined Professionals. *Journal of Counseling and Development, 78,* 293–296.

Crocket, K. (2007). Counselling supervision and the production of professional selves. *British Association for Counselling and Psychotherapy, 7,* 19–25.

Doughty, E. A., & Leddick, G. R. (2007). Gender differences in the supervisory relationship. *Journal of Professional Counseling: Practice, Theory, and Research, 35,* 17–30.

Downs, L. (2000). A literature review of gender issues in supervision: Power differentials and dual relationship. (ERIC Document Reproduction Service No. ED444077).

Falender, C. A., & Shafranske, E. P. (2004). *Clinical supervision: A competency-based approach.* Washington, D.C.: American Psychological Association.

Fall, M., & Sutton, J. (2004). *Clinical supervision: A handbook for practitioners.* Pearson Allyn and Bacon.

Feltham, C. (2000). Counselling supervision: Baselines, problems, and possibilities. In B. L. Lawton & C. Feltham (Eds.), *Taking supervision forward: Enquires and trends in counseling and psychotherapy* (pp. 5–24). London: Sage.

Friedlander, M. L., & Ward, L. G. (1984). Development and validation of the Supervisory Styles Inventory. *Journal of Counseling Psychology, 31,* 541–557.

Gatmon, D., Jackson, D., Koshkarian, L., & Martos-Perry, N. (2001). Exploring ethnic, gender and sexual orientation variables in supervision: Do they really matter? *Journal of Multicultural Counseling and Development, 29,* 102–114.

Granello, D. H. (2003). Influence strategies in the supervisory dyad: An investigation into the effects of gender and age. *Counselor Education and Supervision, 42,* 189–202.

Greenberg, L. S., & Pinsof, W. M. (Eds.). (1986). *The psychotherapeutic process: A research handbook.* New York: Guilford Press.

Greenson, R. R. (1967). *The technique and practice of psychoanalysis* (Vol. 1). New York: International University Press.

Henry, W. P., Strupp, H. H., Butler, S. F., Schacht, T. E., & Binder, J. L. (1993). The effects of training in time-limited dynamic psychotherapy: Changes in therapeutic behavior. *Journal of Consulting and Clinical Psychology, 61,* 434–440.

Hill, C. E., & Lambert, M. J. (2004). Methodological issues in studying psychotherapy process and outcomes. In M. J. Lambert (Ed.), *Bergin and Garfield's handbook of psychotherapy and behavior change* (5th ed., pp. 84–135). New York: Wiley.

Holloway, E. L. (1995). *Clinical supervision: A systems approach.* Thousand Oaks, CA: Sage.

Kraus, D. R., Seligman, D. A., & Jordan, J. R. (2005). Validation of a behavioral health treatment outcome and assessment tool designed for naturalistic settings: The treatment outcome package. *Journal of Clinical Psychology, 61,* 285–314.

Ladany, N., Marotta, S., & Muse-Burke, J. L. (2001). Counselor experience related to complexity of case conceptualization and supervision preference. *Counselor Education and Supervision, 40,* 203–219.

Lambert, M. J. (2007). Presidential address: What we have learned from a decade of research aimed at improving outcome in routine care. *Psychotherapy Research, 17,* 1–14.

Lambert, M. J., & Ogles, B. M. (2004). The efficacy and effectiveness of psychotherapy. In M. J. Lambert (Ed.), *Bergin and Garfield's handbook of psychotherapy and behavioral change* (5th ed., pp. 139–193). New York: Wiley.

Lilienfeld, S. O. (2007). Psychological treatments that cause harm. *Perspectives on Psychological Science, 2,* 53–70.

Llewelyn, S. P. (1988). Psychological therapy as viewed by clients and therapists. *British Journal of Clinical Psychology, 27,* 223–237.

Morgan, M. M., & Sprenkle, D. H. (2007). Toward a common-factor approach to supervision. *Journal of Marital and Family Therapy, 33,* 1–17.

National Association of Social Workers (1999). *Code of ethics.* Washington, DC: Author.

Rapisarda, C. A., & Britton, P. J. (2007). Sanctioned supervision: Voices from the experts. *Journal of Mental Health Counseling, 29,* 81–92.

Russell-Chapin, L. A. (2007). Supervision: An essential for professional counselor development. In J. Gregoire & C. M. Jungers (Eds.), *The counselor's companion: What every beginning counselor needs to know* (pp. 79–80). Mahwah, NJ: Lawrence Erlbaum.

Russell-Chapin, L. A., & Ivey, A. E. (2004). *Your supervised practicum and internship: Field resources for turning theory into action.* Pacific Grove: CA, Brooks/Cole.

Strupp, H. H., & Hadley, S. W. (1985). Negative effects and their determinants. In D. T. Mays & C. M. Franks (Eds.), *Negative outcome in psychotherapy and what to do about it.* (pp. 20–55). New York: Springer.

Thomas, J. T. (2005). Licensing board complaints: Minimizing the impact on the psychologist's defense and clinical practice. *Professional Psychology: Research and Practice, 36,* 426–433.

West, W., & Clark, V. (2004). Learning from a qualitative study into counseling supervision: Listening to supervisor and supervisee. *Counselling and Psychotherapy Research, 4,* 20–26.

Wolberg, L. R. (1967). *The technique of psychotherapy* (2nd ed.). New York: Grune & Stratton.

Ethics in Counseling Supervision

Ethical Supervision Behaviors and Standards of Care

When one goes to any professional as a consumer of services, there is a certain expectation of professional standard of care. Russell-Chapin and Ivey (2004) state, "You expect your chosen expert to have expertise and knowledge in the services you desire. You expect to be treated respectfully and competently" (p. 162). This holds true in the clinical supervision world as well.

Ethical behaviors are typically guided by written organizational mandates adopted by a specific discipline. Of course, ethical codes are designed to protect the consumer, but appropriate ethical codes also protect the supervisor and the profession as well. These documents were written by members of that particular professional organization to assist in providing quality treatment to the client and always doing no harm (Baird, 2002).

For example, the ACES Ethical Guidelines for Counseling Supervisors (2003) address client welfare and rights, program administration role, and supervisory role. These three components all have ethical aspects. Understanding that clinical supervision ethics and ethical behaviors must be the underpinnings of competent supervision is essential.

Corey, Corey, and Callanan (2003) outlined procedural steps to assist supervisees in addressing ethical concerns: identify the problem or dilemma, identify potential issues involved, review relevant codes, know applicable laws and regulations, obtain consultation, consider possible courses of action, look at the consequences of various decisions, and finally decide the best course of action. The authors are not suggesting that these steps must be linear, but the model may be an excellent first method to use in a supervisory session to begin to resolve any ethical issues (Haynes, Corey, & Moulton, 2003). As the ethical dilemmas are presented in the following pages, use the steps outlined above to assist in the reflection anecdotes and resolution of the ethical concerns.

Discussion Question 1

As you read the procedural steps for addressing ethical concerns, identify which step will be the most difficult for you. _____

_____

_____

_____

OVERVIEW

In many respects, there is no more important relationship in the evolution of a developing professional counselor than that of clinical supervisor and supervisee. The clinical supervisor is at the same time a coach, mentor, teacher, evaluator, and role model. Through this complex relationship, the foundation for the counselor's professional values and ethical behavior are formed.

The ethical framework surrounding the supervisor–supervisee relationship provides critically important guidelines for the establishment of a meaningful and respectful professional partnership. By maintaining appropriate boundaries, applying a sound theoretically established supervisory process, and providing essential feedback in a fair, accurate, honest, and respectful manner, the ethical supervisor can be best assured of preparing the supervisee for a successful future as a skilled mental health practitioner (Russell-Chapin & Ivey, 2004).

This chapter will focus on the ethical practice of clinical supervision. Each section will present an ethical problem that could readily arise in any setting where mental health services are provided. The reader will be presented the problem and a set of discussion questions intended to encourage further reflection on the particular ethical issues involved in that situation. Then a short summary of the relevant ethical guidelines will be provided, followed by a suggested course of appropriate action. For purposes of this discussion, the ethical Guidelines of the American Counseling Association (ACA) (2005) will be employed to both guide the authors' analysis of the ethical problem and outline an ethically appropriate course of action. Please note, readers are encouraged to review their own specific professional association's ethical guidelines as they relate to the ethical delivery of clinical supervision. Although the reader will likely find much consistency and overlap, your association's guidelines will be those employed should you need to defend your action in front of a disciplinary review committee, whether that be the American Psychological Association (2002), National Association of Social Workers (1999), American Mental Health Association (2000), or any other professional association and division in which you are a member, such as the Association for Counselor Education and Supervision (ACES) (2003).

Many of the above codes and others may be viewed online through the associations' homepages. Frequently used web addresses are listed in Appendix B. In addition there is a supplemental booklet available through this publisher, entitled *Codes of Ethics for the Helping Professions,* with codes from all helping professions, such as the American Psychological Association, the National Association of Social Workers, and the National Organization for Human Service Education. This 120-page booklet is available to buy for approximately three dollars.

Finally, the chapter will end with a brief discussion of the function of disciplinary review and typical disciplinary consequences of unethical behavior.

GOALS

- Define and identify possible ethical dilemmas and behaviors

- Locate resources for resolutions of ethical concerns

- Understand how counseling supervision ethics frame the supervision relationship

Client Worsens while under the Care of Supervisee

A 16-year-old girl who came to counseling for help with recurrent depression is exhibiting increasingly severe episodes of self-mutilation. The supervisee is very worried and afraid to tell his supervisor about the extent of her self-injury for fear that it will result in a poor evaluation. Eight sessions of counseling have been completed. The client has made vague references to childhood sexual abuse, but to date nothing specific has been addressed in therapy. The supervisee is reluctant to discuss the matter with his client because he is afraid she will become suicidal. The supervisee has not told his supervisor the self-mutilation has worsened.

Discussion Questions 2

1. Should the supervisee keep this information from his supervisor? _____

_____

_____

_____

_____

2. Is this client at risk for suicide? _____

_____

_____

_____

_____

3. Is this case beyond the expertise of the supervisee? _____

_____

_____

_____

_____

4. What might be causing the supervisee's lack of disclosure? _____

_____

_____

_____

_____

_____

5. How can the supervisor monitor the client's welfare? _____

_____

_____

_____

_____

_____

The 2005 American Counseling Association (ACA) ethical guideline that applies to this problem is **F.1.a. Client Welfare,** which states, "A primary obligation of counseling supervisors is to monitor the services provided by other counselors or counselors in training. Counseling supervisors monitor client welfare and supervise clinical performance and professional development."

Possible means available to the supervisor to monitor the services provided by the supervisee are regular meetings with the supervisee, review of client case notes, review of samples of clinical work, and/or live observations of the supervisee's therapy and regular written evaluations, whether in formal or informal formats.

In this case, it is clear the supervisee is struggling but unable or unwilling to disclose his worry to his supervisor. This is not an uncommon supervisee anxiety. Although there may be many problems with supervisee inadequacy and supervisor–supervisee trust, the primary ethical problem for the supervisor is that he does not know that the client is intensifying her self-mutilation. Regular supervision meetings, review of the case record, and videotaped observations of the therapy would likely have brought the matter to the supervisor's attention, where it could be appropriately evaluated and addressed with the supervisee. There are many possible remedies to this case. Perhaps the self-mutilation is increasing due to avoidance of the discussion of her abuse. Perhaps the client is not suicidal, but the supervisee is confusing self-mutilation with suicidal behavior and needs some help making a differential risk assessment. Perhaps therapeutic interventions could be discussed to explore the abuse or to limit the client's self-mutilation. Or maybe this case is too overwhelming for this supervisee at this time, and a referral to another counselor is warranted so that the client's self-harm can be more effectively managed.

Worthen and Lambert (2007) agree that it is time for supervisors to incorporate real-time feedback on client progress, outcome monitoring, and brief client assessments into regular, ongoing supervision. These authors believe it is essential to build in a supervisory outcome management system to ensure that client and supervisees' goals are maximized. In a recent research project, Hannan et al. (2005) asked 48 therapists (22 were licensed and 26 were trainees) to rate their 550 clients for a 3-week period on client progress and client deterioration. These counselors knew that there was a statistical base rate of 8 percent of client deterioration. Even with that information, rarely were they able to predict a negative outcome. Many of the professional therapists were also supervisors. None of the supervisors correctly predicted a negative outcome. The counselors identified 1 of out 40 clients who deteriorated, whereas the computer statistical algorithms identified 77 percent of deteriorated clients.

This subjective optimism may assist us with difficult clients, but it does not do justice and may inhibit therapy progress with high-risk clients (Worthen & Lambert (2007). Garb (2005) also writes that many clinicians prefer their intuitive, subjective impressions to actual statistical data and information. Moving to a more multiperspective system of offering feedback and tracking progress is needed in our clinical supervision world.

Angry Client Wants to End Counseling with Supervisee

A 42-year-old male client is seeking counseling for help with his struggling marriage. He has had repeated affairs but states his interest in wanting to cease his infidelity and recommit to his marriage. He is very nervous about the privacy of his disclosures but is reassured by the supervisee that all of his disclosures are confidential and will not be released to anyone without his written consent. A few weeks into therapy the client becomes very angry after the supervisee tells him he has been talking with his supervisor, Dr. Ellen Smith, about the case and has a good idea how to help him. Unknown to the supervisee, Dr. Ellen Smith is a good friend of the client's wife. The client, now realizing that his counselor's supervisor was Dr. Ellen Smith, becomes very angry and afraid that all he has disclosed will find its way back to his wife. He wants to immediately end therapy with the supervisee.

Discussion Questions 3

1. Did the supervisee sufficiently disclose the limits of confidentiality? _____

_____

_____

_____

_____

_____

2. Does the client have a right to be angry with the counselor? _____

_____

_____

_____

_____

_____

3. Is there risk that this counselor could be sued and/or a complaint brought against the counselor, supervisor, and agency? _____

_____

_____

_____

_____

_____

4. How can the counselor and supervisor best handle this situation? _____

_____

_____

_____

_____

_____

5. What supervisee and supervisor actions could have prevented this problem? _____

_____

_____

_____

_____

_____

The ACA (2005) ethical guideline that applies to this problem is **F.1.c. Informed Consent and Client Rights:** "Supervisors make supervisees aware of the client rights including the protection of client privacy and confidentiality in the counseling relationship. Supervisees provide clients with professional disclosure information and inform them of how the supervision process influences the limits of confidentiality. Supervisees make clients aware of who will have access to records of the counseling relationship and how these records will be used."

The primary mistake made by this supervisee and supervisor is that the client was not "fully" informed as to "specifically" who would see the counseling records. If this had happened, the client may have immediately voiced his concern about the supervisor being a friend of his wife and his worry that his disclosures might find their way back to his wife. This could have enabled the supervisee to address the issues of confidentiality and explain that its protection also extends to her supervisor. Should the client have persisted in his objection, a referral to another therapist with a different supervisor could have been offered. In an article by Kaplan (2003) the author discussed that 80 percent or more of all ethical concerns revolve around the single issue of informed consent. To ensure that clients and supervisees understand all rights, verbal and written consent is essential.

However, in this ethical dilemma the damage has already been done. The client already made what he now perceives as potentially incriminating disclosures. The risk for a lawsuit and/or a disciplinary complaint is high. The supervisee in this situation may be best advised to make a genuine apology for his lack of full informed consent and disclosure of who would have access to the counseling records. The supervisor may also be well advised to offer a similar apology and reassurance to the client that his disclosures are confidential and will not be shared with his wife. This may, in itself, sufficiently reduce the client's anger and worry. If not, the client's anger and mistrust will likely undermine the therapeutic relationship, and a referral to another therapist may be in order.

Although not a factor in the case discussed above, another related issue with regard to informed consent and client rights is disclosure of the supervisee's qualifications and status as a trainee. Many counselors in training are sensitive to a client's perception of their professional competency. Although it may be tempting to avoid this issue with clients, it is the client's right to be aware of her counselor's qualifications and to make an informed decision about who she wants to help her with her concerns. In most cases, clients are more than satisfied working with a counselor in training, finding comfort in the knowledge they are being supervised by an experienced and qualified professional. In those cases where clients do object to a counselor in training, their wishes must be respected, and a referral to a fully qualified professional is appropriate.

Pressure from the Agency to Supervise the New Counseling Intern

A highly skilled, experienced, and licensed professional counselor has been asked by his agency to supervise the new counseling intern from the local University counseling program. None of the other senior agency clinicians are interested in taking on this responsibility but don't want to lose the opportunity afforded them in having the intern help them with the agency's waiting list. The agency director makes a personal appeal to a junior staff person to take on this obligation. Although reluctant and unsure how to provide adequate supervision, the junior staff person accepts the request and agrees to supervise the intern. The two meet on a regular basis, review ongoing cases, clear the agency's waiting list, and generally fulfill the intern's academic requirements.

Discussion Questions 4

1. Is it appropriate for interns to be used to clear an agency's waiting list? _____

_____

_____

_____

_____

2. Does the junior staff person have sufficient experience to supervise the intern? _____

_____

_____

_____

_____

3. Will the intern receive a good experience at this agency? _____

_____

_____

_____

_____

4. Will the clients seen by this intern receive good therapy? _____

_____

_____

_____

_____

_____

5. What special qualifications and training does the junior staff person have to provide the intern with a good supervised experience? _____

_____

_____

_____

_____

_____

The ACA (2005) ethical guideline that applies to this problem is **F.2.a. Counselor Supervision Competence:** "Prior to offering clinical supervision services, counselors are trained in supervision methods and techniques. Counselors who offer clinical supervision regularly pursue continuing education activities including both counseling and supervision topics and skills."

Both the NASW (1999) and APA (2001) ethical standards are also clear on this matter. Working outside of a helping professional's area of expertise may harm clients, supervisees, and the profession.

In the above situation, the junior staff member is likely a well-trained, adequately experienced, and appropriately credentialed counseling professional, but she openly acknowledged reluctance and uncertainty in providing clinical supervision of the intern. In all likelihood, the supervision she provided was adequate, the counseling the clients received was adequate, and the intern had an adequate clinical experience at this agency. However, how might the intern's experience have been enhanced if his supervisor was trained in current supervision methods and techniques? How much better could the intern's clients' therapeutic results have been? And how might the intern's overall clinical experience at this agency have been improved if he had been supervised by a specially trained clinical supervisor? The answer is self-evident. All would have benefited from a far better experience if the foundation of that experience were based upon current standards of competent clinical supervision. Polanski (2000) encourages teaching supervision at the master level and the doctoral level. Courses at the master's level will help trainees to better understand what they need and want out of supervision and assist them in becoming better supervisors at a later developmental stage.

In this situation one might argue that some benefit is better than no benefit at all; after all, waiting-list clients were seen and the intern gained some valuable experience and met his academic requirements, but this is a proverbial "slippery slope." Today's ethical standards require that we provide competent clinical supervision. It might have been more appropriate for the agency to turn down the opportunity for the internship and instead send the junior agency staff member to continuing education on clinical supervision. Or perhaps the junior staff member could have sought supervision on the provision of clinical supervision from an appropriately trained university faculty member, while jointly supervising the intern at her agency. Sometimes real work demands pressure counselors into situations in which they are uncomfortable. Rather than succumbing to demand, it is better to explore your reluctance and take proactive steps at addressing your limited qualifications. Cobia and Boes (2000) go even further by stating that it is the supervisor's responsibility to locate another supervisor who is clinically competent in supervision.

Another issue not addressed in the above situation is competency with multicultural and diversity issues in supervision. Counselors must be aware of and sensitive to the influences of gender, ethnicity, culture, and race in supervisory relationships. As we all likely learned in our basic counseling training, individual differences left misunderstood or misinterpreted can easily undermine rapport, and sidetrack our most well-intentioned efforts. The same applies to clinical supervision. We all bring our personal biases, limited experiences, and stereotypes into every relationship we have. It is incumbent upon each of us to become aware of our limits of perception and to learn how to skillfully and respectfully address these issues as they also inevitably emerge in our supervisory relationships. Kwan (2001) reiterates this philosophy by emphasizing the importance of the counselor knowing him- or herself well. Then and only then will the counselor or supervisor be ready to assist in the supervisee's development.

Using the Multicultural Competency Standards developed by Sue, Arrendo, and McDavis (1992), Kwan (2001) developed the following guidelines to assist helping professionals in exploring personal multicultural journeys. Although these were developed for counselors in training, the same format can be applied to supervisors in training. Read through each sentence, and first decide whether you personally agree or disagree with the guideline. Then reflect on the guideline's meaning. If the guideline is true or useful, then begin to dissect how it might play a role in your work with clients and supervisees.

Attitudes and Beliefs Guidelines

- Culturally skilled counselors believe that cultural self-awareness and sensitivity to one's own cultural heritage is essential.
- Culturally skilled counselors are aware of how their own cultural background and experiences have influenced attitudes, values, and biases about psychological processes.
- Culturally skilled counselors are able to recognize the limits of their multicultural competency and expertise.

Every human being has a culture all to him- or herself. It influences who we are and how life is experienced and handled. This too will definitely impact how we present ourselves in supervision as a supervisee and as a supervisor.

Discussion Question 5

How will working with diverse client populations be a challenge for you as a counselor, supervisee, and supervisor? _____

_____

_____

_____

_____

A Close Friend and Colleague Wants You to Supervise Him

A highly trained and well-respected clinical supervisor, with years of supervisory experience, who has helped many students and professionals fulfill their clinical supervision requirements for their respective professional certification and licensure, has been asked by his friend and colleague to supervise him. It seems that the colleague's graduate counseling education program has now required all faculty to become licensed, and this will require 2 years of clinical supervision. The supervisor, not wanting to disappoint his friend and confidant he can help him, agrees to conduct the supervision. All goes well at first, but as the supervision continues, the supervisor becomes aware of some significant weaknesses in his colleague's approach. He attempts to address these directly with him, but his friend becomes defensive. The supervisor decides to back off. He does not want to hurt their relationship, but the weaknesses become more obvious. The supervisor feels a professional obligation to address it again and attempts to do so. This time his friend becomes angry and demands to terminate supervision. The supervisor, now frustrated and disappointed, agrees that termination may be the best solution. For months thereafter, despite continued efforts by the supervisor to reconnect with his friend, his friend keeps his distance. The supervisor fears the relationship may be forever damaged and remains concerned that his friend has not addressed his weaknesses.

Discussion Questions 6

1. Is it appropriate for a friend and colleague to request supervision from a friend and colleague? _____

_____

_____

_____

_____

2. How should the supervisor have responded to the request?

_____

_____

_____

_____

3. How could the supervisor best deliver the feedback to his friend? _____

_____

_____

_____

_____

4. Is termination of the supervisory relationship an appropriate option? _____

_____

_____

_____

_____

_____

5. What should the supervisor do with his disappointment and continued concern? _____

_____

_____

_____

_____

_____

The ACA (2005) ethical guidelines that best address this problem are **F.3.a. Relationship Boundaries with Supervisees and F.3.d. Close Relatives and Friends:** "Counseling supervisors avoid nonprofessional relationships with current supervisees. If supervisors must assume other professional roles (e.g., clinical and administrative supervisor, instructor) with supervisee, they work to minimize potential conflicts and explain to the supervisee the expectations and responsibilities associated with each role. They do not engage in any form of nonprofessional interaction that may compromise the supervisory relationship. . . . Counseling supervisors avoid accepting close relatives, romantic partners, or friends as supervisees."

The problem above describes a difficult predicament involving collegial loyalty, friendship, and the role of the clinical supervisor. At the outset, all parties seemed satisfied with the arrangement. Although we are not clear whether the supervisor explained to the supervisee the potential conflicts, conflicting roles, and varying expectations across these roles, perhaps such a discussion might have led them to conclude that the arrangement was ill-advised. Having engaged the supervisor–supervisee relationship, they soon ran into trouble. Their friendship became tested when the supervisee rejected supervisory feedback. The eventual consequence was loss of both their friendship and the supervisory relationship. The ethical guidelines clearly state that supervisory relationships with friends should be avoided. The problem involves the difficulty of managing dual relationships and their tendency to undermine one another. Although some dual relationships may be unavoidable, such as administrative supervisor–colleague and supervisor–instructor, others like supervisor and friend are avoidable. Although not an issue in the above example, the ethical guidelines also prohibit sexual relationships between supervisor and supervisee and sexual harassment of supervisees.

Haynes et al. (2003, p. 171) offer several additional questions to help in determining the healthiest decision and resolution of multiple relationship issues.

- Can I explain and justify my decisions regarding supervisees to an ethics board?
- What advice would I give to a colleague who came to me with a similar situation?
- Am I willing for my actions to be public?

A Supervisee's Parent Unexpectedly Dies

A supervisor and supervisee have been meeting for supervision for well over 9 months. During that time the supervisee shared that her mother was ill with cancer. It had been a difficult ordeal for her and a frequent topic in her supervision. The supervisee worked with two clients who were dealing with loss issues, and it was important for her to understand how her own issues were influencing her therapy. Then the personal news came. Her mother had died. The supervisee was very upset and in tears as she informed her supervisor of the news. During their conversation, she asked her supervisor to help her get through the visitation and funeral. The supervisor politely said she could not do so as it would be a breach of supervision ethics for her to have a nonprofessional relationship with her supervisee. The supervisor offered her condolences and scheduled the next supervision session.

Discussion Questions 7

1. Was the topic of her mother's struggle with cancer appropriate content for supervision?

_____

_____

_____

_____

2. Should the supervisee continue to see clients who are also dealing with loss? _____

_____

_____

_____

_____

3. Did the supervisor act ethically in declining the supervisee's request to help her get through the visitation and funeral? _____

_____

_____

_____

4. How else could the supervisor have addressed the supervisee's request? _____

_____

_____

_____

_____

5. What personal feelings might the supervisor be reacting to in declining the supervisee's request? _____

_____

_____

_____

The ACA (2005) ethical guideline that applies to this situation is **F.3.e Potentially Beneficial Relationships**: "Counseling supervisors are aware of the power differential in their relationships with supervisees. If they believe a nonprofessional relationship with a supervisee may be potentially beneficial to the supervisee, they take precautions similar to counselors working with clients. Examples of potentially beneficial interactions or relationships include attending a formal ceremony, hospital visits, providing support in a stressful event, or mutual membership in a professional association, organization, or community."

The supervisor in the above situation was generally acting within her appropriate boundary in citing the ethical guideline prohibiting nonprofessional relationships with supervisees; however, she failed to consider the potentially beneficial relationship she could have established by helping her supervisee get through the visitation and funeral. It seems clear the issue of the supervisee's mother's struggle with cancer had been a frequent topic of their supervision. It is very likely the supervisee found support in the supervisor's therapeutic encouragement while she continued her work with clients who were dealing with their own losses. It may have been very disappointing and potentially damaging to their supervisory relationship for the supervisor to decline the supervisee's request. How will this affect their rapport and the supervisee's sense of trust and future comfort with personal disclosure? It could inhibit it. Perhaps the supervisor had strong personal reasons for declining the request. Maybe she was very uncomfortable with visitations and funerals. Maybe she felt she could not lend much effective support to her supervisee. If these were her feelings, it might have been better for her to have shared them with her supervisee and offered some other means of support. As supervisors we are not immune from our own issues and are powerful role models to our supervisees. In discussing the matter further, the supervisor might have demonstrated how to acknowledge and work through personal shortcomings. Attending the visitation and funeral could have provided an ethically beneficial relationship to the supervisee, but not if the supervisor lacked the confidence or ability to handle it herself.

This ethical dilemma has many unique facets. One issue that is not often addressed is the need for the supervisor to seek counseling and/or ongoing supervision. The importance of supervisors not being counselors at the same time to their supervisees is well documented. There is a fine line to be observed, however. Supervisors have the responsibility in the supervisory process to deal with supervisee's limitations, strengths, and liabilities. There could also be countertransference issues, and those too must be acknowledged in supervision. Much like self-disclosure in counseling, discussing a supervisor's personal issues in an appropriate and relevant manner will not necessarily affect the supervisor–supervisee relationship (Sumerel & Borders, 1996). The authors of this textbook often tell supervisees this rule: "If your self-disclosure feels too good, then you know you have shared too much!" That is when the supervisor needs to seek out counseling and/or supervision.

Supervisee On-the-Job Training

A new practicum student received his placement site notice. He was very excited about the prospect of working at one of the leading private practices in town. His initial interview went very well, and the staff at the private practice offered him the position. The first day on the job, he had four clients to see. He dove right in, did his case notes, and submitted the payment for the sessions to the appropriate office staff. Then his troubles began. He was told he didn't have the clients fill out the correct forms. He didn't properly schedule the next appointments. He failed to collect the right co-pays and deductibles. And worst of all, he didn't inform his clients he was a practicum student and didn't have them sign the appropriate release forms so that a senior staff therapist could supervise his work with them. His first day on the job was a disaster.

Discussion Questions 8

1. Who is responsible for these problems, the supervisee or supervisor? _____

_____

_____

_____

_____

_____

2. What kind of consequence should the supervisee receive? _____

_____

_____

_____

_____

_____

3. How can the problem be remedied? _____

_____

_____

_____

_____

4. What if a client now objects to seeing a practicum student? _____

_____

_____

_____

_____

_____

5. What else does the supervisee need to know? _____

_____

_____

_____

_____

_____

The ACA (2005) ethical guidelines that apply to this situation include: **F.4.a. Informed Consent for Supervision, F.4.b. Emergencies and Absences, and F.4.c. Standards for Supervisees:** "Supervisors are responsible for incorporating into their supervision the principles of informed consent and participation. Supervisors inform supervisees of the policies and procedures to which they are expected to adhere and the mechanisms for due process appeal of individual supervisory actions. Supervisors establish and communicate to supervisees procedures for contacting them or, in their absence, alternative on-call supervision to assist in handing crises. Supervisors make their supervisees aware of professional and ethical standards and legal responsibilities."

In the above example, the new practicum student was given no direction. He had no job orientation, no supervisory orientation, and no briefing on ethical standards and legal responsibilities. He made many mistakes. Although it would have been useful for him to have asked some questions before he agreed to see clients, it would have been better yet if he had had a few hours of practicum orientation. Many graduate programs offer this to students before they are placed in the community, but each placement site is so unique that it should provide its own orientation, complete with an initial supervisory session where expectations, procedures, policies, and appeal mechanisms can be defined. As a consequence of not having this orientation, the new practicum student, the private practice staff, and his supervisor have a mess to clean up. In addition, there is the problem of the uninformed clients who did not realize they were working with a practicum student and didn't understand the supervisory requirements associated with that relationship. Each of them need to be fully informed and offered the opportunity to either continue working with the practicum student or select a new therapist. Each of the problems created by on-the-job training can be repaired, but all of them could have been prevented if the supervisory, graduate school, and placement site responsibilities had been more fully met.

Off on the Wrong Foot and Only Getting Worse

An independent practicing master's level therapist decided she could benefit from ongoing clinical supervision. She developed a list of area practitioners who she felt she could work well with and began the process of interviewing each of them. She hoped to find a highly experienced female clinician with Jungian training. However, after speaking with several prospective supervisors, she couldn't find exactly what she wanted. After some reflection, she decided to contract with a male supervisor who had a psychodynamic orientation. He said he was familiar with Jungian principles and more importantly had provided clinical supervision for over 10 years. Their first supervision session was scheduled for 2 weeks later. The supervisee arrived on time but had to wait 20 minutes before her supervisor finished his last client. The session opened with the supervisor talking about himself, his experience, and his last counseling session. By the time he finished, the hour was over and the supervisee was not able to share anything about her needs and expectations, nor was she able to present a case for feedback. The counselor left the first session worried she had made a mistake in selecting this supervisor but decided to give him another try. As with the previous session, the supervisor was again late. This time he did ask her whether she had a case to present, and she offered a concise client history, diagnostic impression, and questions for supervision. The supervisor listened attentively and then offered his analysis from a psychodynamic, object-relations perspective. The supervisee responded with a puzzled look on her face. She asked, "What symbolism do you think might be represented in the clients dream about an old, gray-haired woman?" The supervisor shrugged his shoulders and asked the supervisee questions about the client's attachment to his mother. The supervisee said nothing. The supervisor then began to postulate about the possible implications of the client's early attachment on his current problems with anxiety. The supervisee respectfully listened but thought, "I've made a terrible mistake in choosing this supervisor. Now what do I do?" Out of courtesy and perhaps avoidance, she agreed to schedule another supervision session but didn't show up. Instead, she wrote the supervisor a letter stating her decision to discontinue their supervision. She explained she really preferred a female supervisor and thanked him for his time.

Discussion Questions 9

1. How specific should a supervisee be in the selection of a supervisor? _____

_____

_____

_____

_____

_____

2. What is the supervisor's responsibility in ensuring a good supervisee–supervisor match?

_____

_____

_____

_____

_____

3. If problems occur, how should they be addressed? _____

_____

_____

_____

_____

_____

4. Did the supervisor have a fair opportunity to adjust his approach? _____

_____

_____

_____

_____

5. Should the supervisee have terminated supervision in the manner she did? _____

_____

_____

_____

_____

The ACA (2005) ethical guideline that is relevant to this problem is **F.4.d. Termination of the Supervisory Relationship:** "Supervisors or supervisees have the right to terminate the supervisory relationship with adequate notice. Reasons for withdrawal are provided to the other party. When cultural, clinical, or professional issues are crucial to the viability of the supervisory relationships, both parties make efforts to resolve these differences. When termination is warranted, supervisors make appropriate referrals to possible alternative supervisors."

The above situation illustrates the confounding problems that evolve from a poor supervisor–supervisee match. The supervisee had some specific expectations for her supervision but contracted for services knowing this supervisor did not meet them. When they ran into problems, the supervisor seemed oblivious to the supervisee's frustration, but neither did she voice her concerns. Instead, the supervisor presumed all was well and the supervisee decided to end the relationship. This too was handled indirectly, with the supervisor thinking it was a gender issue when it appears to have been a professional courtesy and theoretical orientation issue. Although the supervisee was within her rights to terminate the supervision, this was not done after a genuine attempt to discuss and resolve the differences. The supervisor was not given any feedback or offered an opportunity to change his behavior, and he could not give the supervisee an appropriate referral to another supervisor. It would have been better for the supervisee to address the supervisor's tardiness and her dissatisfaction with his theoretical orientation. The termination may still have occurred, but both would have been informed and involved in the process.

You Can't Change What You're Not Aware of

A newly graduated master's degree therapist took a job with an area agency. The therapist arrived with strong recommendations from his graduate program and even stronger recommendations from his internship supervisor. He was given an adequate orientation to his new job and was informed about the performance evaluation process. As the weeks turned into months, the therapist thought he was doing well. Yes, he had made a few mistakes, but these were caught and corrected. Overall, he had the impression all was going well. Then, near the end of his 6-month review period, he was unexpectedly fired. The reasons given were well beyond the mistakes that were previously brought to his attention. They included concern about his attitude, clinical judgment, and ethical decision making. He was shocked and hurt. He had met frequently with his clinical supervisor, but none of these issues were ever brought up. He felt betrayed and angry.

Discussion Questions 10

1. Is it realistic to expect a new professional to make some mistakes? _____

_____

_____

_____

_____

2. Should a counselor be informed of all his shortcomings? _____

_____

_____

_____

_____

3. Is it the supervisor's responsibility to outline corrective action? _____

_____

_____

_____

_____

4. Is it legal for an employer to terminate an employee without disclosure of cause? _____

_____

_____

_____

_____

5. It is ethical for a supervisor to dismiss a counselor without feedback or without referral for reparative measures? _____

_____

_____

_____

_____

The ACA (2005) guideline that relates to this problem is **F.5.a. Evaluation and F.5.b. Limitations.** "Supervisors document and provide supervisees with ongoing performance appraisal and evaluation feedback and schedule periodic formal evaluative sessions throughout the supervisory relationship. Through ongoing evaluation and appraisal, supervisors are aware of the limitations of supervisees that might impede performance. Supervisors assist supervisees in securing remedial assistance when needed. They recommend dismissal from training programs, applied counseling settings, or state or voluntary professional credentialing processes when those supervisees are unable to provide competent professional services."

New professionals are likely to make mistakes. This is generally an opportunity for feedback, education, and further training rather than judgment, punishment, or dismissal. Having said this, all supervisors must oversee and guard the competence of their supervisee's performance. Clients' welfare and institutional liability is at stake. Adequate oversight is best accomplished through a program of frequent review, evaluation, feedback, and documentation. Should remedial work be required, a supervisor is responsible for offering referrals for such assistance. In the above situation, the supervisee was not fully informed of the problems with his performance and was not offered an opportunity to remedy those problems. Should his problems have significantly impaired his therapeutic effectiveness, it may have become necessary for him to be temporarily relieved of his clinical duties. If the incompetence is so severe that after remediation impairment still persists, it is the supervisor's responsibility to see to it that the supervisee is dismissed from his position. These are often very difficult decisions and may require consultation with another supervisor and proper documentation of the rationale for the disciplinary action. In addition, it is important that the supervisee be apprised of his options to address and/or appeal any such decision. Supervision is the primary mechanism by which we ensure clients receive competent therapeutic services. It is also the frontline mechanism whereby clinicians receive the feedback and assistance they need to continue to provide quality service.

From the research by Worthen and Lambert (2007), important contributions may be applied to supervision and training. By providing standardized performance and progress feedback in supervision, counselors in training receive objective and subjective feedback about their skills and treatment. Providing feedback from the client's perspective offers an additional dimension to the feedback. As the authors eloquently stated, "It is the combination of clinical wisdom informed by standardized sources of information that may ultimately contribute to improved outcomes and give us a powerful new focus in supervision" (p. 52).

Counselor Heal Thyself

A graduate professor in a master's degree counseling program supervised several students. She also offered supervision services to community mental health professionals. At times in the course of supervision she became aware of supervisees' unresolved personal matters that seemed to be negatively affecting their clinical work with clients. When this happened with a student, she helped him or her understand the problem and referred the student for personal counseling. She did not want a dual teaching and professional therapy relationship with a student. When this occurred with a community mental health professional, however, she offered the supervisee the opportunity in supervision to work on his or her personal issues. She felt that because she and her professional supervisee already had good rapport and an established financial arrangement, it wasn't much of a stretch to provide both personal counseling and supervision. In addition, her supervision clients seemed to appreciate the convenience of doing both under one roof. All seemed to work well until one case presented a dilemma that neither the supervisee nor supervisor saw coming.

A nonstudent supervisee was working with an older couple and having some difficulty helping them disengage from constant verbal conflict. He tried many different approaches, several suggested by his supervisor, but none were effective. The couple was drifting closer and closer to divorce. The supervisee was very upset by his inability to help this couple. The supervisor recognized this and explored with the counselor why he was so reluctant to accept that perhaps this couple did not want to improve their relationship. During the exploration, the supervisee disclosed that he too was struggling with his marriage. His wife wanted out, whereas he wanted to work on it. The supervisor suggested that this might be the reason it was so difficult for him to accept that his clients might choose to divorce. As they spoke, the supervisee broke into tears and asked his supervisor if she could provide counseling for his wife and him.

The supervisor agreed. They met as a couple for several sessions. Little progress was made. The supervisee's wife still wanted out, and the supervisee didn't want to accept it. As his supervisor tried to help him come to accept that his marriage was ending, the supervisee became very angry and blamed his supervisor for not trying hard enough. The supervisor apologized for being unable to help his supervisee save his marriage, but this didn't stop the supervisee from losing trust and respect for his supervisor. Their supervision was never the same.

Discussion Questions 11

1. Is it reasonable to have one policy about providing counseling to student supervisees and another for private pay supervisees? _____

_____

_____

_____

_____

_____

2. Did the supervisee really need counseling? _____

_____

_____

_____

_____

_____

3. Are rapport and convenience the only factors to consider in agreeing to counsel a supervisee? _____

_____

_____

_____

_____

_____

4. How could this supervisor and supervisee salvage their supervision relationship? _____

_____

_____

_____

_____

5. Why should this supervisor never have agreed to counsel his supervisee? _____

_____

_____

_____

_____

The ACA (2005) ethical guideline that addressed this issue is **F.5.c. Counseling for Supervisees:** "If supervisees request counseling, counseling supervisors provide them with acceptable referrals. Counselors do not provide counseling services to supervisees. Supervisors address interpersonal competencies in terms of the impact of these issues on clients, the supervisory relationship, and professional functioning."

The above situation appears to be advantageous for the supervisee until the counseling fails and the dual role of supervisor and counselor undermine the trust and respect of the supervisory relationship. The supervisor would have been best advised to avoid counseling not only student supervisees but also private pay supervisees. Although it is possible that greed was the supervisor's underlying motive, it is more likely that she was blinded by her well-meaning intention to help the supervisee with his case and his marriage. Sadly, the supervisee lost much more than he likely anticipated. He lost his marriage, therapist, and supervisory relationship. This is an unfortunate example of the serious problem with dual relationships.

Somewhat overshadowed in the above discussion is the issue of the supervisee's need for therapy. It is clear from his struggle with his divorcing clients that this supervisee's difficulty in his own marriage was negatively affecting his therapeutic effectiveness. A referral for counseling does appear warranted. The problem, however, is whether counseling will help him quickly enough to benefit his work with his clients. Or, given his impairment, is this supervisee better advised to refer these clients to another therapist? This is both a difficult and awkward situation to handle, but one an effective supervisor can readily help resolve. This counselor needs to manage his personal issues in such a manner that they do not cause harm to his clients. Should he refuse to get counseling, an ethical problem does exist. Although not an issue in the above problem, should this supervisee remain impaired, the supervisor is obliged not to endorse him for certification, licensure, employment, or in the case of a student, completion of an academic training program. This is one of the hardest boundaries to set with a supervisee, be that person a student or a fellow colleague, but one that is absolutely necessary in order to assure competent professional performance and safeguard client welfare.

Ramos-Sanchez and colleagues (2002) believe in the importance of graduate counseling students seeking out individual therapy. The authors list three areas that may improve through therapy: expanding personal awareness, fostering personal and professional development, and enhancing the supervisory relationship. Haynes et al. (2003) also believe it is appropriate to encourage supervisees to seek counseling. Perhaps if therapy is supported on both ends of the continuum, from schooling to supervision, newly trained professionals will emerge healthier, more confident, and competent.

How Should You Respond to an Ethical Complaint?

It is important to first understand that the primary purpose of a credentialing or licensing review board is consumer protection, and this carries with it obvious legal, professional, and ethical implications. Credentialing boards such as the Center for Credentialing and Education (2001), National Board of Certified Counselors (2003), Approved Clinical Supervisor (2001), and state licensing review boards enforce a set of standards that have been either set forth by a professional organization or put into law by a state legislature. The board's charge is the oversight of the competent provision of professional services. To accomplish this, boards typically review the credentials of all applicants, often require testing of basic professional and practice knowledge, and review and act on any complaints brought forth against any of their certified or licensed providers. Although most professionals understand and accept the value of credential review and testing, the prospect of facing a complaint raises much anxiety.

Complaints can be presented to a review board from many sources, including employers, supervisors, colleagues, and clients. Most ethical guidelines outline a procedure for initial resolution of a complaint through direct discussion with the offending party. In this way, misunderstandings can be resolved quickly, and feedback and corrective action can be immediately taken. However, if the offending behavior is more egregious, the initial attempt at resolution is met with a defensive response, or the inappropriate behavior persists, then a complaint will very likely be filed with a credentialing or licensing review board. The board's responsibility is to then investigate the complaint, determine whether it warrants corrective or disciplinary action, decide what action should be taken, and follow up on compliance with its requirements.

Most complaints brought to a review board are resolved through remediation, requiring additional training or specialized supervision. Other complaints are met with some form of censure, ranging from placement on probation to temporary or permanent loss of a license or certification. This is the source of most practitioners' fear. Will I be reprimanded? Will I be censured? Will I lose my certification or license? Will I be unable to practice my profession? It is no doubt embarrassing and humiliating to be the focus of a complaint, but it is unwise to become defensive and assume the worst.

We are all human beings and as such are capable of making mistakes. Being informed and conscientious about the ethical guidelines of practice and participating in ongoing supervision can go a long way in limiting the potential for complaints. However, should you still become the focus of a complaint, remember that the review board is protecting the consumer and guarding the profession. Be honest in the investigation. Accept responsibility for your actions. Be open to the feedback you receive. If you are given remedial requirements to fulfill, accept them as a learning opportunity and a means to improve your skills. If you are censured, deeply reflect upon your actions and either recommit to your profession and do all that is necessary to reestablish your good standing or accept that this profession may not be for you and refocus on a new career. It is never easy to be the focus of a review board complaint, but it can be a critical and beneficial life-changing experience.

Summary

The challenges of counseling supervision can be best met through the guidance offered by a set of detailed ethical principles for professional conduct. The strongest supervisor–supervisee relationships provide a meaningful and respectful partnership that enhances both professional practice and client care. This chapter reviewed the ACA Ethical Principles as they apply to counselor supervision. These emphasized that a professional counselor's primary responsibility remains the welfare of his clients. All clients should be informed about their counselor's status as a supervisee, and full disclosure should be made as to how the clients' personal information will be shared in supervision. The principles also stated that counseling supervisors should be specially trained and supervised to ensure the quality and effectiveness of their supervision. Conflict of roles and dual relationships should be limited and, if possible, avoided altogether because they have the very real potential of undermining one another. This, however, does not mean that supervisors cannot participate in potentially beneficial relationships with supervisees, such as weddings, funerals, professional meetings, or training seminars.

This chapter also stressed that supervisees should be fully informed of the standards of success, evaluation procedures, job orientation, and any appeal processes that may be in place to challenge an unfair supervisory action. The ACA ethics further recognized that sometimes supervisor–supervisor relationships must be terminated, but this should be done only after attempts to resolve conflicts have failed and both parties have understood and agreed to this remedy. Perhaps most difficult, supervisors should be honest and accurate in their evaluation of supervisee limitations, even if this means the supervisee may not pass a class or fulfill workplace requirements, or may fail to quality for certification and/or licensure. In the case of an impaired supervisee, the supervisee should be referred for remediation (counseling) and not treated by the supervisor, as this will constitute a dual relationship and present a conflict of interest for the supervisor. Finally, this chapter outlined the purpose of certification and licensure review boards and the important charge they have to protect the consumer and guard the profession. Although it is difficult to face a complaint and the possibility of remediation or censure, it is the professional counselor's responsibility to provide competent service and do all she can to bring unethical behavior problems into appropriate ethical compliance.

Chapter Three Final Discussion Questions

1. What are your biggest concerns about entering into a personal counseling relationship?

_____

_____

_____

_____

_____

2. What lessons may be learned if a complaint or grievance is filed against you? _____

_____

_____

_____

_____

_____

_____

References

American Counseling Association. (2005). *ACA code of ethics and standards of practice.* Alexandria, VA: Author.

American Mental Health Counseling Association. (2000). *Code of ethics of the American Mental Health Counseling Association.* Alexandria, VA: Author.

American Psychological Association. (2002). *APA code of ethics and conduct.* Washington, DC: Author.

Approved Clinical Supervisor. (2001). Center for Credentialing and Education. Greensboro, NC: Author.

Association for Counseling Education and Supervision. (2003). *ACES code of ethics for counseling supervision.* Alexandria, VA: Author.

Baird, B. N. (2002). *The internship, practicum, and field placement handbook: A guide for the helping professional* (3rd ed.). Upper Saddle River, NJ: Prentice Hall.

Center for Credentialing and Education. (2001). Greensboro, NC: Author.

Cobia, D. C., & Boes, S. R. (2000). Professional disclosure statements and formal plans for supervision: Two strategies for minimizing the risk of ethical conflicts in post-master's supervision. *Journal of Counseling and Development, 78,* 293–296.

Corey, G., Corey, M. S., & Callanan, P. (2003). *Issues and ethics in the helping professions* (6th ed.). Pacific Grove, CA: Brooks/Cole.

Garb, H. N. (2005). Clinical judgment and decision making. *Annual Review of Clinical Psychology, 55,* 310–323.

Hannan, C., Lambert, M. J., Harmon, C., Nielsen, S. L., Smart, D. W., & Shimokawa, K. (2005). A lab test and algorithms for identifying clients at risk for treatment failure. *Journal of Clinical Psychology/In session, 61,* 1–9.

Haynes, R., Corey, G., & Moulton, P. (2003). *Clinical supervision in the helping professions: A practical guide.* Pacific Grove, CA: Brooks/Cole.

Kaplan, D. (2003). Excellence in ethics. *Counseling Today, 4,* 5.

Kwan, K. K. (2001). Models of racial and ethnic identity development: Delineation of practical implications. *Journal of Mental Health Counseling, 23,* 269–277.

National Association of Social Workers. (1999). *Code of ethics.* NASW Press: Washington, DC: Author.

National Board of Certified Counselors. (2003). Alexandria, VA.

Polanski, P. (2000). Training supervisors at the masters level: Developmental considerations. *ACES Spectrum Newsletter, 61,* 3–5.

Ramos-Sanchez, L., Esnil, G., Goodwin, A., Riggs, S., Touster, L. O., Wright, L. K., et al. (2002). Negative supervisory events: Effects on supervision satisfaction and supervisory alliance. *Professional Psychology, Research and Practice, 33,* 197–202.

Russell-Chapin, L. A., & Ivey, A. E. (2004). *Your supervised practicum and internship: Field resources for turning theory into practice.* Pacific Grove: CA, Brooks/Cole.

Sue, D. W., Arredondo, P., & McDavis, R. J. (1992). Multicultural competencies/standards: A call to the profession. *Journal of Counseling and Development, 70,* 477–486.

Sumerel, M. B., & Borders, L. D. (1996). Addressing personal issues in supervision: Impact on counselors' experience level on various aspects of the supervisory relationship. *Counselor Education and Supervision, 35,* 268–286.

Worthen, V. E., & Lambert, J. (2007). Outcome oriented supervision: Advantages of adding systematic client tracking to supportive consultations. *Counselling and Psychotherapy Research, 7,* 48–53.

Developmental Supervision Models

Common Factors Approach to Supervision

Morgan and Sprenkle (2007) took on the enormous task of looking at the majority of supervision models, theories, and skills in order to identify a common set of supervision practices. From their literature review general supervision constructs were recognized.

- Supervision involves a relationship between a supervisor with greater experience in counseling and a supervisee with lesser experience.

- Supervision involves a structured relationship between the supervisor and supervisee, with the goal of helping the supervisee to gain the attitude, skills, and knowledge to become an effective helping professional.

- Common supervision domains are relevant: development of clinical skills, theories and client dynamics, professional and ethical behaviors, personal growth of the supervisee, autonomy and confidence levels, and monitoring and evaluation of the supervisee.

The literature review produced a first list of 238 supervisor behaviors; after no new activities or domains appeared, the authors developed a three-dimensional approach to supervision, using three continua and four supervisor roles. This newly created conceptual model may assist all supervisors in combining common practices with preferred, specific models.

The first continuum focuses on the supervisory behaviors, from clinical issues and competency in areas such as clinical skills and theories, to professional competency such as personal growth, ethics, and professionalism.

The second continuum emphasizes the various levels of specificity of a supervisor from idiosyncratic/particular on one end of the continuum to nomothetic/general on the other end. It is the supervisor's responsibility to focus on the supervisee's individual needs, the profession's needs, or both. The final and third continuum concerns the supervisory relationship. This continuum is related more to *how* supervisors do their jobs than to *what* they do. This relationship continuum ranges from collaborative on one end of the spectrum to directive on the other end.

The authors summarize their common factors approach to supervision by describing that the content of supervision, the actions of supervisors, and what they do can be illustrated by the first two continua: emphasis and specificity. The final continuum/dimension focuses on the nature of the supervisory relationship. Within these dimensions, four supervisory roles can be seen: coach, teacher, administrator, and mentor.

Morgan and Sprenkle (2007) state, "We are not, therefore, suggesting that supervisors drop their models and merely employ the common factors. Rather, the field is likely to benefit most from a 'both/and' attitude toward specific models and common factors. As has been suggested for clinical common factors, we believe that specific models

OVERVIEW

Before beginning the chapters on different types of supervision models, this chapter will offer a common factors approach to supervision, identifying common elements throughout all supervision models. Then the chapter will provide an overview of developmental models of supervision. Developmental supervision models tend to be flexible based upon the supervisee's needs and outcomes. The basic tenets and stages will be discussed emphasizing supervisee levels of functioning and supervisor's possible interventions and responses. Follow along using the transcription guide in this chapter as you watch the DVD demonstration using a development supervision model. Reflection questions are at the end of the chapter to allow the reader integration of the concepts.

GOALS

- Understand the benefits of a common factors approach to supervision

- Define the needs of each supervisee in differing developmental stages

- Understand the appropriate supervisory response and behaviors of each stage

- Identify when developmental model might be selected for supervision

are the medium through which the common factors work (Sprenkle and Blow, 2004), and which provide the variety and diversity needed to match human complexity" (p. 7).

As the reader continues through the supervision model journey and begins to find the best fit for the supervisor and supervisee, remember to use the common factors approach plus differing supervision models. They are interwoven one with the other.

Discussion Question 1

1. What are the potential benefits of using a common factors approach to better understand the complexity of supervision? _____

_____

_____

_____

_____

Developmental Models of Supervision

The basic tenets formulating developmental models of supervision are that supervisees continue to grow at individual paces with differing needs and differing styles of learning. If this is true, then one of the major goals during developmental supervision is to discover personal needs and focus on whatever it takes to maximize the supervisee's strengths and minimize liabilities. In a study by Hart and Nance (2003), the authors found there is an optimal supervisor style that needs to be used for each supervisee developmental level and/ or need. In other words, there is a certain level of directiveness and support for each development level.

Holloway (1995) writes of at least 18 developmental models. Some examples of different developmental models are Skovholt and Ronnestad (1992), Stoltenberg (1981), and Taibbi (1990). According to these models, in order to manage this developmental nature of learning, the manner in which the supervisee and supervisor interact must also change (Russell-Chapin & Ivey, 2004). As the supervisees mature and grow, their needs and wants from the supervisor will also change. In individual counseling, assessing the developmental level of the client and choosing a corresponding intervention is essential. A similar parallel process occurs within developmental supervision (Russell-Chapin, 2007). Two examples of developmental models will be explored.

Stoltenberg, McNeil, and Delworth's Developmental Supervision Model

Stoltenberg (1981), Stoltenberg and Delworth (1987), and Stoltenberg, McNeil, and Delworth (1998) formulated a developmental supervision model describing distinct levels of supervisees: beginning, intermediate, advanced, and master counselor. During each level or stage, the job of the supervisor would be to structure supervision moving from imitative and demonstrative functions at the beginning level to more competent and self-reliant functions during the advanced levels (Stoltenberg et al., 1998).

In this model a strong emphasis is on the supervisee's ability to better understand self and others, his motivational levels, and his ability to become autonomous. Each level includes those three processes (awareness, motivation, and autonomy), and within each level are nine growth areas to emphasize. See Table 1.1 to better understand each level.

The nine growth areas are intervention, skill competence, assessment techniques, interpersonal assessment, client conceptualization, individual differences, theoretical orientation, treatment goals and plans, and professional ethics. In developmental supervision, the job of the supervisor and supervisee will be to help the supervisee discover personal strengths areas for improvement. This strategy can be a lifelong learning pattern and can be responsible for personal growth throughout a helping profession.

Basic Tenet

- Supervisees grow at individual paces with differing needs and styles of learning often with stages of growth that are dependent upon skill level and need of the client.

When to Use

- Use this model when assessment of the developmental level of the supervisee is needed.

Supervisor's and Supervisee's Roles and Behavior

Levels	Behavior of Supervisee	Behavior of Supervisor
Beginning—Level 1	Little experience; dependent on the supervisor	Models needed skills and behaviors; teacher role
Intermediate—Level 2	Less imitative; strives for independence	Provides some structure but encourages exploration
Advanced—Level 3	More insightful and motivated; more autonomous sharing	Listens and offers suggestions when asked
Master Counselor—Level 4	"Skilled interpersonally, cognitively, and professionally"	Provides collegial and consultative functions

Supervisor's Emphasis and Goals

- Assess the supervisee's developmental level of functioning from levels 1 through 4.
- Understand the supervisee's world, motivational levels, and degree of autonomy.
- Identify needed growth areas in each of the four levels using the nine intervention areas listed below.

Supervisee Growth Areas

- Interventions
- Skill competence
- Assessment techniques
- Interpersonal assessment
- Client conceptualization
- Individual differences
- Theoretical orientation
- Treatment goals and plans
- Professional ethics

Limitations

This model does not go deep enough into specific supervision methods for each supervisee level, and it focuses only on student development as supervisees (Haynes, Corey, & Moulton, 2003). Additionally, in a study of 100 supervisees, Ladany, Marotta, and Muse-Burke (2001) found no differences of supervisees' preferences based on experience levels. The authors write that developmental assumptions may be "based more on clinical lore than on research" (p. 215). Storm, Todd, Sprenkle, and Morgan (2001) found little empirical evidence to support the developmental assumptions.

Discussion Questions 2

1. How might this developmental model assist you as a supervisee? _____

_____

_____

_____

_____

2. How will this developmental model assist you as a supervisor? _____

_____

_____

_____

_____

3. What are your concerns about this developmental supervision model? _____

_____

_____

_____

_____

Hersey, Blanchard, and Johnson's Developmental Supervision Model

Supervisees go through different developmental stages that have different supervisory needs. Loganbill, Hardy, and Delworth (1982) believe it is important to assess these developmental levels, knowing that they may require differing types of supervisory response.

Hersey, Blanchard, and Johnson (2000) expanded that concept, distinguishing four developmental or maturity levels that required four differing styles of supervision: structured, encouraging, coaching, and mentoring. Again for each level of developmental maturity, the supervisor will respond accordingly. In the Maturity Stage 1(M1), the supervisee might tell the supervisor that he doesn't know exactly what to do with this client. An M1 supervisory response may be to explain in structured detail what to do. In the M2 stage, the supervisee may tell the supervisor that she is working with a client and has conceptualized the case like this. An M2 supervisory response is "You have worked hard on this case and thought it out thoroughly; I like how you stated your treatment goals." In the M3 stage, the supervisor is excited to share the details on the case and request additional ideas. An M3 supervisory response may sound like "Using the intentional skill of self-disclosure seemed to work, but have you thought about how it changed the focus of the session?" In the final stage, M4, the supervisee states confidently to the supervisor how the case is developing. The supervisee has very few questions. An M4 supervisory response is "It is fun to share cases and hear how others intervene." (Russell-Chapin & Ivey, 2004).

Basic Tenet

- Just as a client's developmental level is assessed, so must the supervisee's developmental level be assessed, with correlating supervisory responses.

When to Use

- Use this model when the supervisee's comments and questions indicate hints of the supervisee's developmental level.

Supervisor's Role and Behaviors

- The supervisor must assess the maturity level of the supervisee based upon supervisee behaviors and questions. The supervisor responds accordingly with a structured response to a more collegial response based upon need.

Supervisor's Emphasis and Goals

- The supervisor responds to the differing needs and confidence levels.

Supervisee's Growth Areas

- Supervisee's questions and comments will demonstrate growing confidence and corresponding maturity levels.

Limitations

- The depth of this supervision model may be limited. Additional models may be needed to cover all the comprehensive supervision needs.

Discussion Question 3

What words and phrases could indicate M1, M2, M3, and M4 developmental levels?

_____

_____

_____

_____

DVD Supervisory Question

Each supervisee in the DVD demonstration is asked what he or she wants out of the supervision session. Answering the supervision question is the first step in determining which supervision model is needed. This is the supervision question for this chapter: "When my client sabotages the counseling outcome, what additional strategies could I implement?"

Developmental Supervision and the Case of Brad

In supervising Brad, Lori listened to his case presentation, the diagnosis on all five axes, and his supervisory question. The selection of Stoltenberg's (1981) and Stoltenberg, McNeil, and Delworth's Developmental Supervision Model (1987) seemed like a wise fit. Lori first assessed Brad's level of functioning from Level 1 through 4. She looked at Brad's awareness of self and others, his motivation toward the developmental process, and his independent thinking ability. From his supervision question, his ability to articulate the problem, and general skills, Brad seemed to be functioning at Level 4. To offer Brad collegial supervision was easy and very interactive. Lori was able to offer him possible suggestions, and Brad was amenable to many of the ideas.

Transcripts from the Case of Brad

LRC = Dr. Lori Russell-Chapin

B = Brad

LRC: Thank you so much for joining me today.

B: You're welcome.

LRC: I know you've already had three clients today and—

B: Yes, today.

LRC: So, you're just kind of getting me in the middle of all of this, but I really appreciate that. I think what I would like to do, Brad, is start out with your introduction of yourself, please, and tell us a little bit about you, where you are in your career, and then we'll talk about your supervision question and go from there.

B: All right. I have a master's degree in clinical social work from University of Illinois and about 25 years overall counseling experience in various settings. The last 12 years specifically, I have been working in private practice in a private practice setting. I have a clinical social work degree with an occupational social work and mental health background. I have a licensed clinical social worker certification and alcohol and drug abuse as well.

LRC: But why do you continue to still do supervision? I mean, for example, one of the things I mentioned earlier is that when I was on sabbatical last semester, I came back into supervision with your group. I just found it to be so rejuvenating. Why do you continue to do supervision? You've been doing therapy for 25 years now.

B: One is to keep a fresh view. Not to forget tools that I have learned before. Sometimes they get buried in the past and you forget they are in your toolbox. Another is to avoid burnout and have a group setting to kind of detraumatize yourself. Sometimes the trauma of doing therapy is as traumatic as the actual trauma experience the client goes through. It can be passed on that way. So, it gives me a chance to avoid burnout. To maintain, I guess, and keep my skills honed and have an opportunity for the support that deals with difficult cases.

LRC: So, supervision to you is this multifaceted piece of helping stress reduce but also keeping you fresh in your skills?

B: Exactly.

LRC: Well, let's do this then. Brad, why don't you tell me about a case that you find particularly challenging and then, based upon your supervision question, I think I'll pick a supervision stab that might best fit that need.

B: Okay. The client that I am thinking about right now is a 53-year-old married male. He's in his second marriage. However, in the second marriage—actually he was divorced and remarried during that time. He's been on disability since 1993. So, an extended period of time on disability. During that time he's struggled with severe depression, with fairly significant vegetative symptoms, and he's been involved in counseling with a number of different therapists during that time and is currently under the care of a psychiatrist. He actually got referred to me about 2 years ago as a result of his health plan changing under his insurance plan and having to switch therapists because his therapist was no longer involved in his network. He had a pretty good relationship with this person; however, it appeared, at least from his report, that he reached kind of a plateau of progress in their therapy experience. So he decided to seek additional counseling and came in to see me. His presenting issues, in terms of what led him into therapy, seem to be very different from what keeps him in therapy. He's actually started and stopped with me a couple of different times. He talks about his disability and his inability to work because of chronic pain problems as well as the depression. With my background in pain management as well, I thought this would be a good way to kind of turn things around.

LRC: So how long have your been seeing him in supervision—I mean, counseling?

B: Off and on for 2 years now. And when I say off and on, he'll be with me for 3 or 4 months and then he'll take a break and drop out. Cancel or no-show for a session and then come back again and call me later on to get back on track. The most recent episode of counseling—he's been seeing me for about 3 months uninterrupted and has had a couple of no-shows during that time but gets back into it fairly quickly.

LRC: If you had to say—and there's so many cases that you could pick—you have consent from your client as well to talk about him, Brad? Is that correct?

B: Yes. As long as I don't provide identifying information, he has given me consent to permit this discussion.

LRC: Let's call him—Cliff?

B: Cliff is fine.

LRC: Okay. Let's call him Cliff. Based upon his case, Brad, what would be your supervision question?

B: I guess this is a client who tends to sabotage treatment. By that, I mean he shows a great enthusiasm for assistance to resolve a problem but tends to bat down his responses to treatment almost like he is competing against them. So I would be real interested in getting some guidance in terms of additional strategies to address when he tends to sabotage his own involvement in treatment. To keep him on track and give him a more effective outcome. I guess, tied to that—strategies to help him follow through more consistently with the treatment plan goals, including medication management and the strategies we talk about, so he has a more effective outcome.

LRC: Listening to you, Brad, it seems to me that you have tried so many things with Cliff and that you're very action oriented in your therapy. Is that accurate?

B: Yes. I tend to be fairly cognitive and behavioral in my approach and switching focus too.

LRC: Then I think what I would like to do in supervision today is one of the models in supervision called the developmental model of supervision. I gave you a copy of all the different models, Brad, and I am going to run through them very quickly with you, and then we'll really focus on your supervision question.

B: All right.

LRC: But you notice that under the developmental model the basic tenet is that supervisees grow at individual paces, with differing needs and styles of learning. As your supervisor, of course, I would use this when I am really trying to assess your developmental level. This is so easy for me to do with you because you are a master clinician, Brad. As I listen to you—and I have been a supervisor and a supervisee with you, so one of the things that I've noticed is that—I'm going to assess your developmental level, and then I think what I'll do is I'll tell you a little bit about some of the behaviors that I'd be searching for. One of the examples of this would be the Stoltenberg, McNeil, and Delworth developmental model. This came out in about 1992. Basically, you have a beginning level of supervisee, Brad—that would be the brand new novice therapist.

B: Sure.

LRC: You know, my job would be to just model some skills and provide a lot of structure. That is not you. Intermediate Level II: maybe you're striving a little bit more for independence. My job as your supervisor would be to maybe encourage you, to provide you with some inspiration—but you're achieving more independence. That's not you. Advanced Level would be Level III, in which you really are much more autonomous. I would even maybe just listen, but I'd offer suggestions when needed. But you were, Brad, really a great example of this Master Level Counselor IV, which is on the next page. You are so skilled interpersonally. Your conceptualization skills are wonderful, so what I'm doing today is just providing more of a collegial consultant kind of function with you. What I love about that is—you know from consulting—that you don't have to take anything I say, Brad. So that's really nice. If anything I say might be helpful, I think that's great, but you're on such a different level, so I'm really providing supervision from this Mater Counsel Level IV. In each of those levels, though, Brad—and the viewer at some point will have a slide so they can see the same things we're looking at—but there are nine role sessions in each one of these levels. I'm going to go through them very quickly, but the first one is intervention. You really don't need too much about intervention.

B: No.

LRC: Which would be more technical skills. We move into skills. How comfortable are you? Are you intending and can you be intentional with those skills? In a personal assessment, that's really not you. Also, assessment techniques. So you need to know more about testing? That wouldn't be you. But I thought from your supervisor question—this number five, which is client conceptualization—we might still want to do a little client conceptualization with Cliff.

B: I think there's more to understand at this point.

LRC: And just listening, I think I've got some ideas. We can talk about some individual differences between you and Cliff too, Brad. One of the stops I had is that you are so action oriented and, being in supervision with you previously, I also know that you work really hard to try to help your clients change even though you know it's their responsibility.

B: Exactly.

LRC: But I wonder sometimes if—listening about Cliff—if that's not what he really wants to do. I'm not sure he's really convinced that he wants to change yet.

B: Yeah, and that changes from session to session, so it's hard to keep track of what that is.

LRC: Okay. So I thought maybe we could talk about that. Theoretic orientation—it seems to me, you're very adept in changing with the client's needs, so I wouldn't focus on that. We might talk a little about [no.] eight, which is treatment, goals, and plans, and then the ninth growth area is professional ethics. So I think I'll focus on this treatment goal—perhaps individual differences and conceptualization with you. Does that sound okay?

B: It seems that fits what my needs are.

LRC: Okay. Sounds good. If you would repeat one more time, Brad, for me your supervisory question. Please.

B: I guess the first one—these are connected, but the first one is when my client sabotages the process of his own progress in counseling. What strategies can I put in place there to address that, so he has an opportunity to achieve a better outcome in terms of his own expectations for therapy? And this goes back to the fact that his goals tend to change from one session to the next. In terms of really understanding what he is wanting out of counseling. The other is to identify strategies for change that might hook him into the counseling process and be a little bit more committed in following through in the things that he even agrees with during sessions that he thinks would be appropriate interventions to address his concerns but often doesn't follow through with outside of the therapy process.

LRC: And again, we are just providing a Master Level IV kind of collegial bouncing things back and fourth, Brad. One of the things that became really evident with me with Cliff was that you said he has this chronic neck pain. Kind of neck pain—

R: Neck and shoulder pain. Yes.

LRC: And that I think dealing with him on kind of an abstract metaphor level might be really fun. So I was wondering if you could share with me what do you think the function is and just your opinion of neck pain and shoulder pain. I'm looking for maybe symbolism. I'm looking for physical connections, but what would you say that pain might offer him?

B: During the course of our counseling together and exploring his disability, that's actually gone through a couple of revisions in understanding it. The first one was simply a consequence of his job. His job responsibility was basically to observe train cars switching back and forth, and turning his head from left to right during every 8-hour shift all day. A very responsible job. It was a lot of stress. Very similar to an air traffic controller in terms of responsibility. And my first approach, and his approach was simply a consequence of that. However, being on disability this long and the fact that he continues to experience chronic pain even when he is not doing that work, it took on a different meaning. At one point in time, it seemed to be tied to his own view of his disability in general and whether or not he actually had a personal goal to get off of it. Within the last three sessions, he began to talk about feeling frightened, and he was actually going to get healthy and have to go back and work again.

LRC: Get healthy? Wow.

B: So, maybe metaphorically it's a way to hold him in place so he doesn't have to accept responsibility for the changes that may be involved if he heals and goes back to work. It also seems to be connected in terms of his view of himself. His self-esteem, his self-image, is very low. He views the rest of the world as looking at him as a pain.

LRC: Oh, really? That's interesting, isn't it?

B: He talks to me about how each person he is in a relationship with tends to view him as a burden or a pain of some kind.

LRC: Well, I think that's fascinating because I was thinking about the neck and shoulder pain. That somehow it's a disconnect between what I think in my head and my feelings.

B: And the rest of his problems.

LRC: Yeah. Exactly. So I wondered where that was headed with him is that—you know, "I'm too afraid, I have this giant responsibility. I'm not sure I really want to do this." So I wonder if that chronic pain—he has to have it because if he doesn't have it anymore, it's the old miracle question kind of thing: "What would happen if you suddenly lost this pain?" He would have to go back to work, I guess.

B: Yes.

LRC: And maybe the issue is, is it possible that he doesn't want to be a railroad engineer anymore? Can he find some other thing so that he doesn't have to have that pain and be a pain?

B: Combined with his preoccupation with pain is a very negative view of himself in terms of his own confidence level. We have explored a resistance to job change, whether or not that's what his resistance is. He talks about it as something that he can do that's fairly easy. He describes it as a job that doesn't demand much of him and says it's the only thing he is qualified for. So an expiration and just beginning to open dialogue around "What else would you do if you could do anything you wanted to do, if we just opened the parameters without any restrictions?" We even have him fantasize about the desk job. He begins that process and then switches away from it very quickly basically by challenging or rationalizing any option as being a poor one.

LRC: That's so interesting because I think that metaphor piece about disconnection is—what I sense from Cliff is that he is almost like wrapping a large cocoon around himself to keep him safe. A distance from everyone in his life. And I don't know, Brad, because you're so good with imagery, but what would happen, you know, in a cocoon when one transforms? And I wonder—

B: Metamorphose.

LRC: Yeah. I wonder if somehow Cliff could examine the transforming in metamorphosing into whatever he wants so be. Which would be not pain.

B: I think using imagery with him in that very abstract way may put him in a position where he's actually more comfortable exploring the idea than just intellectualizing it and discussing it with him more directly. So that is something that I will have to try with him.

LRC: And it may not work, but I just wonder as I listen to you talk if that would work. The other thing you told me, Brad, that I thought was fascinating about Cliff was that you had mentioned in your case presentation, in his house they're trying to move. Is that correct? Closer to his wife's job?

B: Actually, in the last session they actually sold their house and have found a house that they have put a deposit on.

LRC: So, he is moving. I mean, literally.

B: Movement is happening. He actually cancelled his last session because he had panic attacks around getting notice from the real estate agent that there were a number of repairs that would have to be done to his home before they could move, and he saw this as another curse on his life.

LRC: Sure.

B: You know, what would appear to be a fairly routine experience for most people going through home sales, kind of fixing up a few things to get ready for if it sells, has turned him into another very weak person again. Just someone who can't handle the stress.

LRC: "I just can't, so this—." Well, what I had thought about was the fact that their moving is so interesting, but you had mentioned that he had come to you a couple times and said that he had ghosts in his house.

B: Yes.

LRC: Could you tell me more about the ghosts? There were two characters—I remember something about that.

B: Yeah.

LRC: Were there two different ghosts?

B: He's actually determined that there's a bad ghost, or an evil ghost, and just a fun-loving, happy-go-lucky ghost. Before this house was put up for sale and before they were deciding to move to get closer to his wife's job, the dialogue of these ghosts would often come at the very end of the session. He would drop them in my lap right before he was walking out the door. And you're talking about how bad life is and that they would get involved in his routine work around the house. He said that once he believed that they had tried to trip him up with a garden hose. Another time he thought that they had thrown the extension cord into the hedge clippers in front of him, so he cut it in two. And at the time he was getting ready to sell his home, he was believing that one of the ghosts was trying to sabotage their ability to sell their house, because something that he had repaired 3 months before broke down 20 minutes before they were to give their house a walk-through. To show it to somebody who was looking at it.

LRC: So, Cliff has these external things in his mind that are hindering his progress, and I bet you've done this, Brad, so I'd just be curious to know this. I think it would be great fun to befriend those ghosts. Have you had conservations with Cliff and the ghosts?

B: We've talked about the ghosts, but we haven't actually had him process or do anything directly with the ghosts in terms of identifying what role they play in his life.

LRC: Because here's—I think, the connection between the cocoon, that imagery of the cocoon, and that transformation thing—which is I wonder if there's not really a ghost in Cliff who is fun. Like he actually sounds like he could be some fun, prankish kind of thing, and then there's that kind of nasty, evil kind of ghost. If you processed that, do you think he could come to the part that, as he transforms, those are the different parts of who he might be?

B: I think that this is a great opportunity to actually explore the impact of why he's projecting that part of himself in anything.

LRC: Yeah.

B: Projects himself in all his relationships in a negative way, and this would be a chance to kind of see how he projects himself into that particular experience with the ghosts.

LRC: Because I think, Brad, that there is sort of a theme again. That there's this transformation that's occurring—however, very slowly—and that it feels like these other pieces he shares with you, it's like, "I'm going to tell you about a ghost, and this guy's going to think I'm so nuts, he won't ever work with me." But I think if we befriended them, then he could be—as you said, begin to see, "Oh, maybe there's this part of me that's maybe prankish and fun. This part of me that's maybe detrimental to my progress." So, I can see this theme of his transformation occurring. My other piece, Brad, as I listen to you talk, is you've tried so many things with Cliff, and this is the piece I was wondering about, to answer your supervision question, which is what if—because you are so action oriented as a therapist and what I know of you as a person—if Cliff senses that from you, Brad, and says, "Brad, I'm not ready to move that fast." Is there anything to that?

B: Well, this has come up repeatedly during the course of counseling in terms of his resistance and exploring that and talking about it with him. And so I went from being very direct in the therapy process and action oriented with him to that becoming second to the role of counseling and leaving it up to him from one session to the next.

LRC: Um, okay.

B: With the expectation that he would drop out of counseling, and again resist even that, because he projects a desire for you to give him solutions so that he can knock them down and prove to you how they're not going to work.

LRC: And how you can't help him.

B: So stepping out of that role leaves him kind of baffled about what to do next because he's wanting something he can disprove. So by stepping out of that role, there have been a couple breaks in counseling. One of the breaks occurred following that, I guess, redirection and letting him know that he'll be responsible for setting the goals for the session and kind of focusing on where he wants to go with this. And then he would come back for a couple of weeks and that was it. And then he calls me back and says, "I'm ready to work. I want to take a look at this stuff. I want to address it."

LRC: Really.

B: So it appears, at least where we are now in terms of the dance, that he does that long enough to get me to hook back into the process with him so that he can get empathy from the process of therapy with me. He seems to be looking for someone to say and agree with everything that he's experiencing in terms of his life and to say, "That's an accurate view. That negative view is accurate"—that his pessimism is accurate. And so stepping into that role with him and giving him empathy temporarily in the process and asking where he wants to go now with this is kind of a dance. We keep going back and forth.

LRC: I love your word though, Brad. I think the word "dance" is probably accurate. That sometimes you lead and sometimes he leads, but it seems like right now you are allowing him to process at his own pace. Which, I think, Brad, knowing what I know about you, must drive you crazy. Does it?

B: It requires a lot of patience. Yes, it does.

LRC: It must require a lot of patience on your part.

B: But it gets more and more intriguing in terms of—you know, in terms of wanting to understand him and see if there is a way to unhook this dance.

LRC: What a great lesson to know that as you as a counselor allow him to grow at his own pace—although it takes much patience for you—that he does transform. I mean, it sounds like he's starting to gradually grow and—I don't know. You said he's not very receptive to medications but that you've been working really hard to get him off medication.

B: The medications I've been trying to get him off of are the painkillers and the narcotics. The ones that are obviously addicting. He's also very inconsistent with medications that we think would be helpful—the psychiatrist and I think would be helpful in his progress. And he's very somatic in his focus so that if he experiences any difficult sensations or sources of stress, his knee-jerk reaction is to address those with medications. He'll change his medications back and forth, and if he hangs on to some that have actually been discontinued, he might switch back to those again from one session to the next.

LRC: This is a really tough question. I'm just asking the question, Brad. Do you like him? Do you like Cliff?

B: Yes, I do. I actually like him a lot.

LRC: Okay. Because, see, I think Cliff is coming to you saying, "Don't like me. I'm going to give you everything I can throw at you so you won't like me. So you will go away like everybody else in my life." Is that possible? Do you think he's testing you?

B: That may be part of the dance. That he can't actually let go of it until he's got a response that he's expecting. And since I haven't been giving him that response, because of the unconditionality of the process, maybe that keeps him coming back to physically prove me wrong.

LRC: Because it feels as if he is beginning to trust you. Even though it's been this long arduous process of a couple years, it feels like he's started to trust you and finally is saying, "Hey, maybe I can symbolically be okay and have that pain somewhat go away." And he's actually moving—physically moving houses. I find that amazing. And it would be fascinating to me, Brad, if we ever get to talk about this in supervision again, will the ghosts follow him?

B: I would expect. I would predict that they will.

LRC: Isn't that interesting? That's fascinating. Anything else, Brad, that you want to discuss in our time together today that we haven't hit upon, perhaps?

B: The preoccupation with the somatic issues in terms of his pain, chronic pain issues, and the ghost and the cocoon and the negative view of self are all kind of wrapped in with an even bigger area of his life. It has to do with avoidance as a wooden personality. I think, to know the clue to the dance that we have in our relationship is that he's only really letting one other person into his life right now and that's his wife. It's kind of a love–hate relationship because he doesn't like being dependent and he also doesn't like her being dependent on him, and they both have a significant amount of somaticism in their relationship. In both her and his interpersonal interactions with each other. I think there's a driving force for him to continue coming back to me because there's somebody fresh to kind of go through his medication with. I don't think his wife is real sensitive to his experience. I think she's kind of detached.

LRC: Jaded, from that point of view.

B: Yeah, and she's desensitized to it. She doesn't give him that validation. But he's so avoiding. He doesn't allow anyone else in his life. He doesn't build other relationships. He doesn't follow through on any of the things we do in regard to direction for building a social network or support system for himself.

LRC: But it sounds like you've tried to do that, Brad, but that maybe that last piece of this whole process, which is "I have to expand my social circle out. I can't just have you and my wife. There have to be other people. Perhaps a job and all those kind of things."

B: A job or even staying within disability but building a support system outside of that in his life.

LRC: What a fascinating case, Brad. Well, I guess I'll go backward then. You gave me two supervision questions. What have you—what will you take from supervision today? And before you answer that, I'd like to have you go backward and give me your multiaxial diagnosis, Brad, if you could.

B: Sure.

LRC: On Axis I, what is the presenting symptom?

B: Under Axis I, I got three different, I guess, merging diagnoses: major depressive disorder. Recurrent. It's very severe. I say without psychotic features, but there have been occasions with these illusions, including the ghosts, that you wonder if there are some psychotic aspects to that. Dysthymic disorder. He has lot of unresolved depressive issues associated with family of origin, extended family, and even his own children that are just kind of mild level, but more personality-based symptoms of his depression.

And a panic disorder. His anxiety management process is very poor, and he tends to work himself up to a pretty significant level of panic. It also feeds back into his depression and hopelessness that goes along with that. Under Axis II, he scores very high on the assessment techniques. He scores very high on avoidant personality disorder and mixed personality disorder with depressive features, dependent, negative, and passive-aggressive features on that scale.

LRC: And the Millon validated your impressions in the beginning?

B: I wondered about borderline for a while, and he actually doesn't score very high on that, but all of the other symptoms flying out regarding passive-aggressive natures—it's really hard to differentiate sometimes. Under the Axis III, which is the medical, he has problems with TMJ in terms of chronically grinding his jaw. Fibromyalgia. Chronic neck and shoulder pains that have been on the medical side is his disability along with his chronic depression.

LRC: I think that's interesting too, though, Brad—that's the piece that I had forgotten about—the job—because that's that same piece of "I just can't say what I need to say. I just can't get it out," you know, and he just keeps it all in. That's that disconnect between mind and body again too. That's fascinating. And Axis IV, the psychosocial stresses?

B: Serious financial problems, obviously, with disability and him and his wife both having chronic medical problems. It puts him in a financial stress. They also have very poor boundaries, so they are involved in rescuing and taking care of children who make poor choices and bailing them out constantly. So, financial concerns are very difficult, with a recent bankruptcy. There's also moderate-level stress associated with relocating and going through a complete change in terms of living situation. His Global Assessment of Functioning has ranged with me from 40–50, but never higher than that.

LRC: No higher than 50?

B: Right now it's probably more of a 40.

LRC: And so, based upon that GAF, you're saying he's struggling. He's not really functioning.

B: Can't maintain a job.

LRC: Yeah. But he is working. It does sound that he does come—when he comes, Brad, he's working in counseling. Occasionally.

B: At times. Yes. It's very cyclic.

LRC: Okay. Well, based upon what you and I talked about today in supervision, what will you leave with today, Brad, that might help you continue with Cliff?

B: I guess, one is kind of refocus and be aware of the dance that I'm involved in with this client and how many of my issues are being pushed into the relationship in terms of the action-oriented focus rather than allowing him to move at his own pace. I guess I've been aware of that process and have been trying to manage it, but I think I can be a little bit more aware of that. The use of metaphor, I think, is one that I haven't expanded on in this particular client situation a whole lot. I think we've touched on it at times, but I get wrapped up or kind of sidetracked by his pessimism even in discussion of metaphor. And so sometimes I get dropped off the side, but I think if I stuck with that and if I took him down that path a little bit further and had him explore that, it might open him up to be able to discuss his fears more comfortably.

LRC: Yeah, because he'd be maybe sitting away from it a little bit, to a degree.

B: His primary defense against his fear is his pessimism and negativism. Basically, if can shoot it down, he doesn't have to deal with it.

LRC: Well, you know, as I listen to this talk in this collegial kind of consultant fashion, the Carl Jung statement of if, you know, if something is not working, don't keep doing it. I think that I love maybe the idea that the imagery might take him to a different place. I really like that. I appreciate you, Brad—your willingness to know that sometimes we just want clients to change so badly, but they're not ready to do that, and that this is going to be a slow and arduous process; but what a fascinating person. And how lucky is he to have you, Brad, because you care about him and you like him, and I don't know if he has that many people in his life who like him.

B: At this time he's trying to make sure that's the case.

LRC: Yeah. Well, I'm sure. I'm glad. I think he's moving. Literally and figuratively. I thank you so much, Brad. I know how busy you are, and I love being in supervision with you as my supervisor when we do our group supervisions, so thank you so much for working with me today.

B: I appreciate the chance too.

LRC: Oh, you're welcome, Brad. Thank you.

Summary

The developmental models have similarities and differences from other models. As the reader continues with each supervision model, look for those concepts that are unique and some that are common. Continue to discover which models seem to best fit the supervisors', supervisees', and clients' needs. You may find that each model has something to offer supervisors and your supervisees. Remember that developmental models allow the supervisor to respond flexibly, depending where the supervisee's needs are, and offer specific supervisee interventions for each level of functioning.

Chapter Four Final Discussion Questions

1. Based on Brad's supervisory question and his case presentation, why did Lori select the Stoltenberg, McNeal, and Delworth Development Supervision Model for this supervision session? Review the chapter for possible reasons. _____

_____

_____

_____

_____

2. What are the strengths of this model for a supervisor? _____

_____

_____

_____

_____

_____

3. What are the strengths of the developmental model as a supervisee? _____

_____

_____

_____

_____

4. When do you think a developmental supervision model will best serve you? _____

_____

_____

_____

_____

References

Hart, G. M., & Nance, D. (2003). Styles of counselor supervision as perceived by and supervisors and supervisees. *Counselor Education and Supervision, 43*, 146–158.

Haynes, R., Corey, G., & Moulton, P. (2003). *Clinical supervision in the helping professions: A practical guide.* Pacific Grove, CA: Brooks/Cole.

Hersey, P., Blanchard, K., & Johnson, D. (2000). *Management of Organizational Behavior: Leading Human Resources* (8th ed.). Upper Saddle River: NJ: Prentice Hall.

Holloway, E. L. (1995). *Clinical supervision: A systems approach.* Thousand Oaks: CA, Sage.

Ladany, N., Marotta, S., & Muse-Burke, J. L. (2001). Counselor experience related to complexity of case conceptualization and supervision preference. *Counselor Education and Supervision, 40*, 203–219.

Loganbill, C., Hardy, E., & Delworth, U. (1982). Supervision: A conceptual model. *The Counseling Psychologist, 10*, 3–42.

Morgan, M. M. & Sprenkle, D. H. (2007). Toward a common-factors approach to supervision. *Journal of Marital and Family Therapy, 33*, 1–17.

Russell-Chapin, L. A. (2007). Supervision: An essential for professional counselor development. In J. Gregoire & C. M. Jungers (Eds.), *The counselor's companion: What every beginning counselor needs to know* (pp. 79–80). Mahwah, NJ: Lawrence Erlbaum.

Russell-Chapin, L. A., & Ivey, A. E. (2004). *Your supervised practicum and internship: Field resources for turning theory into action.* Pacific Grove: CA, Brooks/Cole.

Skovholt, T. M., & Ronnestad, M. H. (1992). *The evolving professional self: Stages and themes in therapists and counselor development.* Chichester, England: Wiley.

Sprenkle, D. H., & Blow, A. J. (2004). Common factors and our sacred models. *Journal of Marital and Family Therapy, 30*, 113–129.

Stoltenberg, C. D. (1981). Approaching supervision from a developmental perspective: The counselor-complexity model. *Journal of Counseling Psychology, 28*, 59–65.

Stoltenberg, C. D., & Delworth, U. (1987). *Supervising counselors and therapists.* San Francisco, CA: Jossey-Bass.

Stoltenberg, C. D., McNeil, B. W., & Delworth, U. (1998). *IDM supervision: An integrated developmental model for supervising counselors and therapists.* San Francisco: Jossey-Bass.

Storm, C. L., Todd, T. C., Sprenkle, D. H., & Morgan, M. M. (2001). Gaps between MFT supervision assumptions and common practice: Suggest best practices. *Journal of Marital and Family Therapy, 27,* 227–239.

Taibbi, R. (1990). Integrated family therapy: A model for supervision. *Families in Society, 71,* 542–549.

Theoretical Specific Supervision Models

Theoretical Specific Supervision

Theoretical specific, or psychotherapy-based, supervision uses the tenets, constructs, and theories developed for counseling and change to assist supervisors with supervision. Therefore, there may be as many theoretical specific supervision models as there are counseling theories.

Helping professionals who adhere to a specific school of thought and therapy (cognitive-behavioral, psychodynamic, Rogerian, etc.) believe that naturally it may be wise to supervise from that same theoretical orientation. In the earliest period of supervision, competent therapists became the supervisors of new trainees. There was little formal training or coursework for supervisors, so at that time clinicians *had* to apply their belief systems to supervision (White & Russell, 1995). The major advantage to the supervisor and supervisee is that if they share the same theoretical orientation, it maximizes the modeling that can occur in supervision (Bernard & Goodyear, 1998). The supervisor can demonstrate discipline-specific skills as well as integrate necessary theoretical constructs.

A disadvantage may be that the supervisor is not familiar or comfortable enough with a needed counseling theory to model it. If so, consultation with an expert is required. Another possible liability may be that one theory is too limiting in focus. Also, what constitutes change in counseling may not be the same in supervision.

There are too many theoretical specific supervision models to mention them all. Five theoretical supervision models will be examined for our purposes here.

Discussion Question 1

When would you want supervision to be conducted using a theoretical specific supervision model? _____

_____

_____

_____

_____

_____

OVERVIEW

This chapter focuses on the advantages and disadvantages of using theoretical specific supervision models. The supervisor needs to be familiar with the chosen counseling theory in order to assist the supervisee in expanding technical skills. Five different psychotherapy-based supervision models will be illustrated. Again use the transcription in this chapter as you watch the DVD demonstration using a psychodynamic supervision model.

GOALS

- Familiarize supervisors and supervisees of the strengths and liabilities of theoretical specific supervision models
- Assist supervisees with possible personal concerns that may interfere with the counseling and supervision process using discipline-specific constructs

Woods and Ellis's Rational Emotive Behavioral Supervision Model

If a supervisor viewed *Rational Emotive Behavioral Therapy (REBT)* as the favored theoretical orientation, two main skills would be required during supervision. First, the supervisor would have to identify the problem and irrational thinking of both the supervisee and the client. Then the supervisee and supervisor would select ways to dispute and challenge those same irrational thoughts as a method for changing and learning new, productive thoughts and behaviors (Ellis, 1989; Woods & Ellis, 1996). A key objective in cognitive behavioral supervision is teaching cognitive behavioral techniques and correcting misconceptions about cognitive behavioral counseling with clients and supervisees (Liese & Beck, 1997). Behavioral and cognitive behavioral supervisors will emphasize and expect the supervisee to demonstrate more technical mastery than most supervisors (Bernard and Goodyear, 1998). For further information on cognitive behavioral supervision, peruse the materials from Woods and Ellis (1996) and Liese and Beck (1997).

Basic Tenet

- The main premise of REBT supervision is to help the supervisee challenge and dispute any irrational thoughts that may be interfering in the counseling and supervision process.

When to Use

- REBT supervision is recommended when there is a need for expansion of knowledge of theory and its techniques.
- Continuity and modeling, especially in the area of distorted thinking on the part of the supervisee, is required.

Supervisor's Roles and Behaviors

- The supervisor's main role is to provide active and direct supervision in accordance with REBT tenets and interventions.
- The supervisor needs to help the supervisee master REBT skills and theoretical understanding.

Supervisor's Emphasis and Goals

- The main goal is technical mastery, but not supervisory relationship.

Supervisee Growth Areas

- The supervisee will begin to see and hear irrational personal and client thoughts that interfere with change.

Limitations

- Probably the major limitation of REBT supervision and all theoretical specific supervision is the narrow focus. The focus, on one hand, may strengthen theoretical skills, but it may also be so specific that the theory excludes other essential components that may well be beneficial to the client and supervisee (Russell-Chapin, 2007; Holloway, 1995).

Discussion Questions 2

1. What would be the most difficult aspect for you as a supervisor or supervisee using REBT supervision?_____

_____

_____

_____

_____

_____

_____

2. As a supervisor, what strategies could you employ to help supervisees work through irrational thoughts? _____

_____

_____

_____

_____

_____

_____

Rogerian Person-Centered Supervision Model

Using supervision from *person-centered theory*, the supervisor would ensure that the basic facilitative conditions were in process throughout the supervision session. Emphasis would be on unconditional positive regard, building trust, and creating a genuine environment for the supervisee to express self-doubts and fears about confidence in personal counseling skills (Hackney & Goodyear, 1984; Rogers, 1961). The evaluation aspect of supervision is not a main emphasis in person-centered supervision, and Lambers (2000) states that the only agenda is to be fully present and allow the supervisee to be open to the experience with the client. The supervisee's growth potential and self-actualization are the main focus (Haynes, Corey, & Moulton, 2003). For additional information on person-centered supervision, read Patterson (1997) and Lambers (2000).

Basic Tenet

■ The main tenet is to provide the necessary facilitative conditions for the supervisee to grow and develop into the counselor he or she may become.

When to Use

- Rogerian supervision is selected when the supervisee needs and wants to better understand the experience of the client.

Supervisor's Roles and Behaviors

- The relationship is essential in Rogerian supervision.
- Nondirective active listening skills are necessary.
- Providing an atmosphere of unconditional positive regard is a foundational element.
- Evaluation is not a critical factor, only the growth of the supervisee as measured by personal insight.

Supervisor's Emphasis and Goals

- The main goal is the supervisee's growth and the better understanding of the client's perspective.

Supervisee Growth Area

- Building personal confidence and self-understanding in the counseling process is the main area of growth.

Limitations

- Although creating a supervisory atmosphere of safety and trust is helpful to a supervisee, some supervisees may struggle with this nondirective environment. During the early stages in a counseling career, the skill and confidence level may not be secure enough for self-exploration.

Discussion Questions 3

1. As a supervisor or supervisee, what frustrations might you incur using Rogerian supervision? _____

_____

_____

_____

2. What might the supervisee need to self-actualize? _____

_____

_____

_____

Bradley and Gould's Psychodynamic Supervision Model

In *psychodynamic supervision*, additional emphasis may be on parallel process (Doehrmann, 1976). Parallel process is the dynamic that occurs in the client–therapist relationship that is played out in the supervisee–supervisor relationship. The supervisor may focus on the resistance that the supervisee had during the session and investigate what resistance the supervisee may have toward the supervisor. Bradley and Gould (2001) believe that the main goal is to focus on both the intrapersonal and interpersonal dynamics of the supervisee's relationship with everyone, whether they are clients, colleagues, friends, or family. The textbook authors find that psychodynamic supervision may also assist supervisees to make the unconscious conscious, allowing them more freedom of choice in counseling and personal living.

Another psychodynamic theory that may assist a supervisee and supervisor is object relationship theory (Goldstein, 2001). Walsh (2009) writes, "Object relationship has two meanings. The first meaning focuses on the quality of our interpersonal relationships. The second focus is on the internalized attitudes towards self and others" (pp. 62–63). Helping the supervisee realize those internalized attitudes and "the power of the situation in the person" (p.131) may assist the supervisee in better understanding the dynamics created between the client–counselor and supervisee–supervisor. In psychodynamic supervision, understanding object relationships is essential, as the major goal is to identify the main roles of relationships in the client's life and the supervisee's life. For more in-depth information on psychodynamic supervision, read Frawley-O'Dea and Sarnat (2001), Haynes et al. (2003), and Walsh (2009).

Basic Tenet

- The basic tenet in psychodynamic supervision is the examination of intrapersonal and interpersonal relationships and the parallel process that plays out during the client–counselor interaction and the supervisee–supervisor experience.

When to Use

- Psychodynamic supervision may be selected when the supervisee seems to be "stuck" in the counseling process and shows signs of attraction or dislike for a particular client.

Supervisor's Roles and Behaviors

- The supervisor may work on the main constructs of psychodynamic theory such as resistance, transference, and countertransference displayed throughout the counseling and supervision sessions.

Supervisor's Emphasis and Goals

- The supervisor's main goal is to focus on the supervisee's interpersonal and intrapersonal conflicts in counseling and the supervision process.
- Struggles and patterns with clients, colleagues, supervisors, and family may be explored.

Supervisee Growth Areas

- A primary growth area is the intrapersonal growth of the supervisee.
- Examining possible unconscious motivations underlying counseling choices allows the supervisee more freedom of choice in later counseling and supervision sessions.

Limitations

- If psychodynamic supervision is the only supervision of choice, the supervisee may grow intrapersonally, but not technically.

Discussion Questions 4

1. How might your own family-of-origin issues hinder working with the client, supervisee, or supervisor? _____

_____

_____

_____

_____

2. What kinds of transference and countertransference concerns may inhibit your supervisory process? _____

_____

_____

_____

_____

_____

Pistole and Fitch's Attachment Theory Supervision Model

Attachment theory in supervision can be especially helpful when the focus is on the supervisory working alliance (Pistole & Fitch, 2008). In Bowlby's (1988) attachment theory, the author provides a clear understanding of relational bonding, motivation, affect management, and actions that are pertinent to the supervisor–supervisee relationship. Ladany, Friedlander, and Nelson (2005) identify two essential components in the supervisor–supervisee relationship: the quality of the emotional bond and the supervisor's astuteness to the supervisee's needs (Pistole & Fitch, 2008). It is the supervisor's responsibility to be aware and sensitive to the supervisee's "vulnerability and need for support and reassurance" (Ladany et al., 2005, p. 13). A useful attachment supervision intervention is that of supervisee critical incident. Discussing these personal experiences such as deaths, divorce, and so on, can activate the attachment system and assist in creating a healthier working alliance. If additional information on attachment theory is warranted, review the works of Mikulincer and Shaver (2007).

Basic Tenet

- The main tenet in the attachment supervision model is focus on the importance of the therapeutic and supervisory working alliances.

When to Use

- The attachment supervision model is used when the supervisee may be struggling with issues of bonding and motivation.

Supervisor's Roles and Behaviors

- The supervisor has an active role in providing interventions that assist the supervisee in discovering awareness concerning the supervisory process.

Supervisor's Emphasis and Goals

- The main goal is for the supervisor to reassure and encourage the supervisee when counseling and supervision become stressful and awkward.

Supervisee Growth Areas

- The supervisee will gain insight and safety throughout the supervision process. This will allow the supervisee to better understand personal attachment patterns that may cloud counseling and supervision outcomes.

Limitations

- The focus may be too specific as to allow for counseling growth in all areas of counseling and supervision.

Discussion Questions 5

1. Who in your life has provided the most support for you? How does that impact you? As a supervisor? As a supervisee? _____

_____

_____

_____

_____

2. From your own history, to whom have you attached, and who has abandoned and neglected you? How does that impact your working alliances with others? _____

_____

_____

_____

_____

3. What is the pivotal or critical incident in your life that has influenced how you look at relationships in general? _____

_____

_____

_____

_____

Prouty's Feminist Theory Supervision Model

Feminist theory of supervision offers an added depth to supervision and its relationships by emphasizing collaborative and equal partnerships between the supervisor and the supervisee (Prouty, 2001; Morgan & Sprenkle, 2007). The supervisory process and expectations are clearly defined, which increases the odds for supervisee participation (Corey, 2001). Haynes et al. (2003) state, "Although the supervisory relationship cannot be entirely equal, the supervisor shares power in the relationship by creating a collaborative partnership with supervisees. For example, instead of the supervisor providing specific direction to the supervisee, the supervisor can help the supervisee think about his or her clients in new ways, formulate interpretations and devise interventions" (p. 122). In Prouty's 2001 research, five feminist concerns were acknowledged as central features in supervision: gender issues, power inequalities, the role of affect, diversity concerns, and socialization skills. For additional readings on feminist-based supervision, see Prouty, Thomas, Johnson, and Long (2001) and Carta-Falsa and Anderson (2001).

Basic Tenet

- The main tenet involved in feminist supervision is to work together as a supervisory team to collaborate on important supervisory issues.

When to Use

- Feminist supervision is utilized when diversity understanding and power inequities need to be addressed.

Supervisor's Roles and Behaviors

- The supervisor's role is that of equal partner in the supervisory process.

Supervisor's Emphasis and Goals

- The main goal is to eliminate the power differential between the supervisee and the supervisor. This equity allows for less insecurity on the supervisee's part and additional opportunities for independence and safety.

Supervisee Growth Areas

- The supervisee begins to appreciate personal power by asserting supervisory needs and wants.

Limitations

■ The feminist supervision model adds an essential layer to supervision by focusing on power, oppression, and diversity concerns. However, all aspects of counseling competency need to be addressed to ensure supervision efficacy.

Discussion Questions 6

1. How may your beliefs about gender roles influence the way you interact in supervision?

_____

_____

_____

_____

_____

2. What would it look like during a supervision session if there were power equity between supervisor and supervisee? _____

_____

_____

_____

_____

_____

DVD Supervisory Question

The supervisory question is the foundation for selection of a supervision model. This chapter's supervision question from this supervisee was "How can I best approach my client's invitation to hear him sing at a Battle of the Bands?"

Theoretical Specific Supervision and the Case of Julie

Again, when conducting supervision with Julie, one of the first things Lori did was listening to her supervision question. She selected psychodynamic theory because as Julie expanded her concerns, her fears tended to focus around some possible countertransference needs. Lori chose psychodynamic supervision and tried to adhere to its tenets throughout the supervisory process. In psychodynamic supervision, additional emphasis may be on parallel process (Doehrmann, 1976). The definition of parallel process is the dynamic that occurs in the client–therapist relationship is played out in the supervisee–supervisor relationship. As Julie's supervisor, Lori needed to focus on any resistance that Julie and her client had during the session and investigate what resistance she may have toward the supervisor.

DVD Transcripts from the Case of Julie

LRC = Lori Russell-Chapin

J = Julie

LRC: Julie, thank you so much for joining me today, I appreciate it. I know how busy you are.

LRC: No problem.

LRC: What I would like to do to get us started is have you introduce yourself, if you would. Tell us a little bit about you, where you're working, what you're doing. And then we'll talk about supervision.

J: Okay. My name is Julie Roth. I'm 27, I'm doing my internship at the Antioch Group in Peoria, Illinois, and I will be graduating in May with my master's in Human Development Counseling, agency track.

LRC: And after you graduate then, Julie, you'll be licensed for your first year of counselor licensure?

J: Correct. And I'll be working to get my LCPC afterwards.

LRC: Very exciting time. So, thank you for coming in because I know how busy you are. Are you also studying for your comprehensive exams?

J: Yes.

LRC: So, thank you very much for coming in. So, tell me a little bit about this case that you're seeking supervision for.

J: Okay, my client is 18 years old; he lives with his mother and his brother, who's older. His parents have been divorced for many years and both parents have remarried. His mother since has been divorced, but she still has—oh boy, she now has a boyfriend. My client originally came to me with a presenting problem of depression in conjunction with the relational problems with his mom and his then girlfriend. And so we've been working a little bit though the girlfriend to address some relational issues with his mom, and his depression seems to have lightened up a little bit. He is much more hopeful now.

LRC: Good. Give me your multiaxial diagnoses, if you could please. You're welcome to look. Please do.

J: Okay. Thank you. Axis I: Diagnosis of 296.22, which is major depressive disorder. Single episode. Moderate. V61.20, which is a parent–child relational problem. There is no diagnosis for Axis II.

LRC: Let me stop for a second. So, no diagnosis—meaning, "I don't believe he has a personality disorder?"

J: Correct.

LRC: But there has been no assessment?

J: Correct.

LRC: Okay.

J: And nothing on Axis III. He is a pretty healthy guy. Axis IV: His mom has a new boyfriend, and he recently broke up with his girlfriend, so—goes with the psychosocial issues. Axis V, his global assessment of functioning, is current at his last session, which is between mild and moderate symptoms.

LRC: So he is functioning okay. He's doing fairly well, but he brings to you these relationship issues.

J: Yes.

LRC: What would be your supervisory question then that you'd ask of me?

J: Well, I guess just counseling the actual relationship as well. There seem to be some transference and countertransference issues that may be popping up, and I think I was hesitant to maybe address those, and so now I'm a little hesitant and nervous on how to address them directly with him.

LRC: It seems to me that—I had a chance to watch the counseling tape—and it seems to me, Julie, that there was one specific question that he asked you toward the end of this tape where you just—which is unlike you—but you just stopped talking. You just kind of went—and your eyes got really big and you stopped talking. What was the question he asked you?

J: My client is in a band, he plays bass, and he just mentioned that he would love me to attend one of his upcoming concerts. It's a Battle of the Bands. And he wrote a song and he had ended up going to be playing it. And so he said, you know, I should really be there.

LRC: So he would like you to attend?

J: Yeah.

LRC: And that's what made you stop and you just sat up?

J: I had no idea how to respond because in my mind I was thinking, okay, my ethics class, you know—what would be the correct way to respond? But then at the same time, how do I want to respond?

LRC: So, you were—it created great dissonance for you.

J: Yes.

LRC: It was a real dilemma. Well, let me tell what I, based on your question and your concerns about transference and countertransference—I think the model of supervision, Julie, that I'll use is a theoretic-specific model of supervision. If you had to say—and I'll have you look at your paper in just a second—if you had to say—what main orientation, counseling orientation, theoretic orientation, were you using with Steven?

J: I probably would say more psychoanalytic. We've tried cognitive behavioral in the past, and he was very good with that, but he's also very intelligent, and so when we talk more about going into themes and patterns, he's very responsive to that.

LRC: And because I've seen so many of your counseling tapes, Julie, I wouldn't say this is the orientation that you typically use. Is that accurate?

J: Yeah.

LRC: So there was something with Steven that said, "I need to change and go in a different direction."

J: Uh-huh.

LRC: All right. Let's take a look at this model that I handed you, this information, Julie, and I'll just share it with you. The viewers can see this online, so in just a second they'll see this. The basic tenet of the theoretic specific model is that the supervisee's benefit from a supervision process focuses on the same theoretical orientation being practiced in counseling. So if I choose to use this today with you, then it will pretty much focus on the same thing that you did with Steven. Does that part make sense?

J: Yeah.

LRC: I think when I've used that is when I'd say, I want to choose this model because for some reason there needs to be an expansion of that skill base for you. And that there may be something going on with you that's either inhibiting something going on in the counseling process or perhaps we need to make it grow in a better direction.

There could be many in the multitudes of models; the Rogerian if you were Rogers, RBT if you were using rationally motivated therapy, or you said—you mentioned cognitive behavioral at one point. I think what I would like to do is maybe this psychodynamic model a little with you today. And so, my role will be to provide you supervision in basic accordance with psychoanalytic theory.

J: Uh-huh.

LRC: And so here's what I'm going to focus on, Julie, I think today. This is based upon your supervision question. I think I'd like to focus on your relationships, because you said he came to you with issues of relationship with him. In psychoanalytic supervision, it says that possibly there's a parallel process. That what's happening in counseling will probably be happening in supervision or other issues in your life.

J: Okay.

LRC: So, the basic thing that I'll deal with today is resistance. And I watched the tape with Steven and I saw him resisting you. He would look away from you. He would change the subject so there was some resistance, and I'll see if you agree with that. I want to talk a little about transference and countertransference, and then we'll keep doing this parallel process through the entire supervision today.

J: Okay.

LRC: Does that sound like it might be where you want to go?

J: Yeah, it sounds good.

LRC: Okay. And so again your question is "How can I best approach Steven's invitation to hear him sing at this Battle of the Bands?"

J: Right.

LRC: All right. Well, let's do that. I guess what I'd want to know, Julie, is a little bit about—you told me he has some issues with his mom.

J: Uh-huh.

LRC: And by the way, do you have consent to have us show this tape down the road and also to talk about Steven?

J: Yes.

LRC: Is it written and—?

J: Yeah. He's good.

LRC: Okay. Good. I think what I'd like to do is you said he has issues with his mom?

J: Uh-huh.

LRC: I would like to talk to you a little bit about maybe a therapeutic mom, Julie. Because I think it will go into this issue of relationships for you. Tell me about what it will mean to you—and I know you recently got married.

J: Yes.

LRC: Congratulations.

J: Thank you.

LRC: What will it mean for you to be a mom someday?

J: It will be a tremendous joy and honor, I think. I think that—I guess in part it will fill a part that I don't even know is empty right now. I look forward to it. I'm not ready for it yet, with all my schoolwork and career. But I think it will be fun. I look forward to having a rowdy home with all the kids running around.

LRC: So there's lots of them, huh?

J: Yeah. And it not being quiet—it just not being—not like yelling but everyone around the dinner table—each having their own chores.

LRC: Chatting and…

J: Yep. Exactly. Just fun.

LRC: Well, you said something that is really fascinating, Julie. You said, "Well, I'm not ready to be a mom yet because I have a lot of things going on." According to this model, it may suggest, Julie, that you're not ready to be what's called a therapeutic mom either.

J: Okay.

LRC: And I wonder if, going back to that look on your face, that the viewers will get to see it at some point, but it was like—

J: Deer in headlights?

LRC: It was like a deer-in-the-headlights kind of thing. It really was. I wonder if some of it might be that you're afraid to be a therapeutic mom. When I say that to you, tell me what that resonates? What do you think about that?

J: I think I agree and disagree.

LRC: Okay.

J: I didn't realize that was a role I could take, I think. So when he said that, and I responded in such a "oh my gosh, what am I supposed to do?" way, I really didn't know what I was supposed to do, and I think in terms of a therapeutic mom I didn't realize that there's some safety in that. That it was, I guess, effective? And that it would benefit the client. So, I guess that probably I was steering away from that, not wanting to cross any boundaries or do anything that might lead the client to become somewhat dependent.

LRC: Uh-huh. So, it had something to do with—first of all, you weren't even sure that you could go there.

J: Uh-huh.

LRC: And then you said, "I'm not sure I'd be effective at it."

J: Uh-huh.

LRC: Well, tell me about that piece. What makes you think you might not be effective at it, Julie?

J: It's very—I guess, there's no clear-cut role.

LRC: That is absolutely true. I am with you there. One hundred percent.

J: So as a new counselor, it's kind of tricky. How far can I go? And I guess I should just trust my gut, but no one talks about the gut in textbooks—it's all . . .

LRC: No, they don't talk about that intuitive piece of it.

J: No. Not at all. And so I guess I'm learning now that I have to trust that, and if I sense that a client needs something or can benefit from it, just go with it rather than worrying about if it would be effective. Because then I'm focusing on myself rather than the client.

LRC: So, you could see maybe, if there is such a thing—just throwing it out—there is such a thing as a therapeutic mom, that maybe you could go there and maybe it might be all right to go there.

J: Uh-huh.

LRC: If you went there, Julie—and talk to me a little, but from a therapeutic mom—and Steven says, "Would you come, come and see me play at this Battle of the Bands?" Rather than thinking he might be hitting on you—I mean, is that part of what you thought? That maybe he was—maybe he has a crush on you and that's the transference piece. Maybe he does have—I mean, we didn't even go there—maybe he does have a crush on you, Julie.

J: I guess for me, again, it's the yes and no. I don't want to admit that I think that he might have a crush, and then I also don't want to maybe believe that he has a crush.

LRC: Okay. Stop there. Let's go there for a second. Why would that be bad? If he had a crush on you?

J: I wouldn't know how to respond to it.

LRC: And so if you trusted your intuition though—and what do you know about that, Julie? Let's just say, what do you know about process therapy and immediacy in counseling?

J: Oh, this is so rich. We could talk about it and it's not only for me, but we—I think both would benefit in our relationship: counselee and counselor.

LRC: That's the transference from client to you. Talk to me a little bit about—and we'll get back to therapeutic mom in a second—talk to me about countertransference from you to Steven. And go back to "Has there been a time in my life when someone I know has talked to me or asked me out and I didn't want to go there?" Does that ring any bells to you?

J: Absolutely.

LRC: You have a smile on your face.

J: I've never really known how to address that, I guess. I've always tried to be polite and never really thought of what I wanted. I'd always respond with how I thought the other person would want to be responded to.

LRC: Wow. And how would that hinder the therapeutic process if you only responded to your client the way you think they would want to be heard?

J: Tons. One, I might be misreading it completely, so it might not be what they're thinking at all. And two, if it was what they're thinking, it may not be what they need. It may not be what would be the best for them or for their counseling relationship.

LRC: Uh-huh. And so anything you take to this counseling relationship—that's what you told me Steven's problem was, he could talk about relationships, he could learn about relationships with you. Right?

J: Yeah.

LRC: In a therapeutic environment, in a safe therapeutic environment—and he might—not only will you learn about relationships, but Steven will certainly be able to relate better to women?

J: Absolutely.

LRC: Moms? Girlfriends that he breaks up with? And so if there's any resistance, Julie, anywhere—I thought maybe Steven had some resistance—where do you think the resistance is coming from?

J: Actually, I probably think it's coming from me. He does look away a lot, but that tends to be his style, I think. I think it's probably from me.

LRC: Maybe. That's possible. And Julie, I want to say to you, don't be afraid of it. You said it well: "It's going to be rich." If you can go there—and you might be wrong, I might be wrong, and he'll say, "I feel silly." But, find out. And again, whatever your client gives you, you can use.

J: So this is where resistance is nerve-racking for me.

LRC: It is. Tell me more about why it's nerve-racking.

J: I have no idea of what I'm going to come across, and in counseling it's fine because it's what the other—it's the client issues and whatever they throw at me usually is fine.

But when it comes to my stuff, you know, I have no idea of what he is going to say and how it might relate to whatever countertransference I'm dealing with.

LRC: Let's go back to this whole thing of self-disclosure because you would be doing some self-disclosing at some point. What do you know about self-disclosure, Julie? In counseling?

J: Well, that it can be incredibly effective when done properly, when—if it's for the client's benefit. Like when you said several times in class, "If I feel oh so good afterwards and the client just kind of sits there and really doesn't have a reaction, then it probably was for my benefit rather than the client's, which would be inappropriate."

LRC: Absolutely. So it could be rich. I love the word, Julie. It really could be rich, and it doesn't have to take up a lot of time, but then you don't have to be afraid of it anymore. I think that you've been afraid of it.

J: Absolutely.

LRC: I do think that deer-in-the-headlights thing was definitely there, and so I think what you could do is provide that environment and teach him how to deal with things. Like rejection, perhaps, or "No." If a client says that to you again, you could say, "I'm really flattered. Thank you so much, but I think what we should be is just concentrate on things in here."

J: Uh-huh.

LRC: But now I'm going to switch gears and go into therapeutic mom again. We've got all that other thing out of the way.

J: Yeah.

LRC: Let's just say, though, that it truly is that he needs a therapeutic mom, Julie.

J: Uh-huh.

LRC: What would a mom do when their son has written a song and is performing it with the Battle of the Bands? And he's had lots of rejection in past.

J: I would hope she would go.

LRC: Why do you want—how come you want her to go?

J: Well, I mean, the mother would be there and be supporting to him and she would not necessarily agree or like the song or the style or anything like that, but by going to the Battle of the Bands is accepting him as he is and the interest that he has. And I think it models love.

LRC: Models love. It shows him how to make a connection. It shows him how to ask for something and he may get it. He might ask for something and he may not get it. So now we've got to talk all these different levels, Julie. So therapeutically, you may see some benefit to being his therapeutic mom. But now how do you make sure that he knows that this is therapeutic mom going to a concert? What kinds of things can you do to safeguard that?

J: I think we can just bring that out in the open.

LRC: Yeah. And you can bring it out in the open and say, you know, "That might be something I could do, and maybe my husband and I will join you." And why might that piece be important?

J: I think that would be incredibly important. One, it's providing a model of a healthy relationship, which he doesn't really have between two people who love each other in that romantic way. But it's also reminding him that I have a life outside of the counseling sessions that we have, and that I'm taken. I married. So I just don't have to worry about that.

LRC: Exactly. And setting boundaries. "Yes, I'm willing to go. I'm clarifying, saying this is what I can do." So, Julie, you need to know that what we've discussed here today is honestly very controversial. A lot of people disagree with it.

J: Okay.

LRC: But I guess what I'm wanting you to do is—as you learn all your counseling theories and techniques and you get into process therapy, which is one of your strengths that we've been working on in class, that you sometimes do have to trust your intuition. Something you've felt. So if we—and when the viewers get to see your tape and they see the deer-in-the-headlights kind of thing, I think it would be really fun for you to replay that in your head. Let's just do that very quickly here. Let's say that Steven says, "I have a poem and it's being turned into music, and I'm going to play it at a Battle of Bands, and I'd really like you to come." What could you do, Julie?

J: The deer comes out again. I think I would take the safe route. I think I would say, "I'm so flattered. Thank you. I look forward to you bringing it to the next session on CD, but I don't know if it would be . . . ." See, this is where it stumbles me. I don't want to say it would be inappropriate, but I don't want to say it would be unethical, because it's not necessarily that.

LRC: How about this. Let's do this. You be Steven and you ask me to come to the— hold the dynamics. I'm old and 50 and you're young and cute. I mean, let's just play this out a little, but . . .

J: Okay.

LRC: You be Steven and I'm Julie.

J: Yeah, and I created a song and we're going to be playing it, and I think you should be there.

LRC: So, you would like me to go to the Battle of the Bands?

J: Yeah.

LRC: Wow. I've never heard, Steven, you ask me to do anything like that. It sounds like it's important to you.

J: Yeah. And I'm not really sure why because it's not like I'm going to be asking just anybody.

LRC: Uh-huh.

J: Cuz you're my counselor, but I really don't know why I'm asking.

LRC: Well, guess with me. I mean, you can't be wrong. We've already gone through all this, Steven. So you can't be wrong. Just guess. Why do you think you'd like me to go to the Battle of the Bands?

J: I think . . . Well, I like when you're proud of me, and so I guess I kind of want to show you what I can do, and you would be able to hear my songs too. What I was going through when I wrote it.

LRC: So, let's go back a little bit, Steven. You said something really important. You said, "I'd like you to be there and I'd like you to be proud of me." Again, tell me how come it's important that I'm proud of you.

J: Because I really don't feel like a lot of people are proud of me.

LRC: And somehow you feel like the relationship we have here is "I care about you"? Is that what you're saying? And that, I'd be proud of you if I saw what you did?

J: Yes.

LRC: Steven, I know this is hard but, you know, this is great. I think we've done a good job in our therapeutic relationship, and I do care about you and I would like to hear you play. But I want to make sure that there's nothing else there. That, for example, maybe my husband and I could go. What would you think if I brought my husband?

J: That would be fine.

LRC: I don't know this, but I wonder sometimes if—because I'm young and I'm female—if sometimes I really make you uncomfortable, Steven?

J: It's really uncomfortable now.

LRC: You're really uncomfortable now? Well, I just think we should talk about anything. I don't know this for sure, but I just wonder if maybe you're putting more into our relationship than therapeutic. Tell me about that. I know it's uncomfortable, but tell me a little bit about that.

J: I don't know. I flirt with all girls. It's just how I respond.

LRC: Okay. So that's how you respond to everyone. Well, you know, you say you're flirting with me then?

J: I wouldn't say that, but maybe I am.

LRC: Okay. Maybe just a little. Well, I'm flattered, but I think there's another piece that I can provide you and maybe that's a different kind of friend. I think I can support you, but you don't have to flirt with me, and I think there's two ways we could do this. Maybe I could ask my spouse if he would like to go to the Battle of the Bands. We could hear you. Or, Steven, the other thing we could do is you could bring your poem and music in and we could hear it here. Tell me, which direction are you headed?

J: I don't—I guess we could bring it in because we've listened to music in here before, but I don't know. It would be different. It's not just me. It's the whole band and the atmosphere, and you would be there.

LRC: So it would provide you—it's not just listening to music in here. It would provide you with a—first of all, I would understand a lot more, right? But it would provide you with a kind of different setting, having me be there too. Okay. Well, let me do some thinking about it, Steven. I'm not sure I know yet if that's the best answer. I want you to think about it too, and then how about if we talk about this at our next counseling session. Then we'll talk more about that.

J: Okay.

LRC: That sound okay?

J: Okay.

LRC: All right, Julie. Thank you for letting me do that. Now, tell me what any of that felt like for you.

J: Oh, it was good actually.

LRC: What was good about it?

J: Well, the modeling. I guess I really didn't know what path to take and what to be with it. Again, it's just going through the process, the processing process, and I guess not getting caught up, as the counselor, with the topic. Dealing with it like I would with anything that he might throw.

LRC: Uh-huh. Oh, but Julie, you just said something really important that you said earlier: "You know, I can usually take whatever my clients give me, but this piece is so different for me." And I think what you're learning is how to deal with this personal part in counseling. Counseling is very intimate.

J: Yes.

LRC: It's one of the most intimate things I can think that we do.

J: Okay.

LRC: And so as you grow as a counselor, this is a piece that you are going to have to learn how to do. Even though it's maybe uncomfortable. That was the word that you used.

J: It is uncomfortable.

LRC: And if there's a parallel process, if there's a parallel process between counseling and supervision in life, you know, sometimes it's uncomfortable. So Julie, let me do one other thing with you, and then I'm going to close today with asking you what you gained out of this supervision session. There might be a parallel process between—according to the literature—counseling and client and also supervision. Tell me what's going on between us. What do you think happens between us in supervision? I think I'll give you a little bit of self-disclosure. I think oftentimes you think that I know always what I'm doing in therapy.

J: I'd say yes and no—I'm really good at those yeses and nos. I think that I don't think that you always know what you're doing.

LRC: Uh-huh.

J: But I think that you always know where to go.

LRC: Exactly. Because I don't have the answers, but I've been doing this long enough to know that I have to go to a certain resource to get there.

J: Exactly.

LRC: And so sometimes, Julie, I parallel process. I think you need to know that I don't always have the answers. And once you know that, you can quit searching in counseling for you to know all the answers.

J: Uh-huh.

LRC: Because I certainly don't have all the answers. I do oftentimes know where to go to get the resources. I think I told you the other day that I've gone back into supervision. That I'm now a supervisee as well as a supervisor, and that's another valuable resource for me. So, I'm hoping that once you leave the program, Julie, that you will continue to do supervision because it's so valuable. But I wondered if there might be some of that parallel processing happening between us too, as a supervisee?

J: I highly respect you. I don't think that you are perfect by any means.

LRC: Well, that's good because, boy, that relieves a huge burden because I'm not.

J: But I highly respect you. I appreciate your genuineness and I think that I appreciate the modeling that you do, so in a way maybe I view you as a therapeutic mom or supervisory mom.

LRC: Well, how interesting. Isn't that interesting?

J: Yeah.

LRC: Yeah.

J: Because I think moms model, and effective moms, you know, are highly respected, I think, by their children, whether it's when they're kids or adults.

LRC: And even when sometimes they don't like what their mom has to say.

J: Yeah.

LRC: Absolutely. And so, Julie, I really want you to think about that. I think that piece is just very valuable. That things do happen in supervision that happen in counseling that happen in real life. And so I guess I'll end today with asking you, what did you get out of supervision today? We spent time on this theoretic-specific model, so what did you glean out of supervision today?

J: I think that I'm learning my style a little bit, and I really don't know what the title is, but to trust my instincts and to go with my gut. And if I'm nervous to go with my gut, to definitely, one, bring it to supervision, and two, ultimately I need to bring it into the counseling process, not for myself but just to use it as a process in self-disclosure. Because I do believe in the transference/countertransference, and I would hate— I don't think it's a bad thing by any means—but I think it would impede the relationship from growing if it's not handled.

LRC: Uh-huh. Absolutely.

J: So I took that. I also—that I'm going to have to get some guts to deal with the personal stuff. I do agree that it's quite intimate, and I think that really what I'm learning and what I took from today is how to balance the professional piece and the personal piece and how to be genuine and professional at the same time. I think before there was always like a straight line in my mind that, you know, I can be firm and genuine and life loving.

LRC: Yes.

J: But then when I put my counselor hat on or whatever—when I have to be professional, almost like stand up straighter.

LRC: And never the two shall meet, right?

J: Right.

LRC: And that just doesn't happen, Julie.

J: It's just kind of becoming that, where I can be both roles. It's a little painful.

LRC: I think it is painful, isn't it? It's scary and it's painful.

J: Yeah, but it's fun.

LRC: But I also think, Julie, there's this piece of resistance there—that if you believe in resistance, that resistance is—I always view resistance as healthy. Resistance from you as well as from the client as well as from a supervisee or supervisor, because it tells you that that person is strong enough to deal with what you have to deal with. And so if Steven has some resistance to you, know that that's okay. He's saying, "Wait a second. I want you to deal with me gently, but I'm okay. I've got the ego strength. I can take it." And so just remember, I believe it's a healthy thing. Now, some people don't even believe in resistance. Some people don't believe in countertransference, Julie, or transference. I think, as you said, your going is sometimes painful, but you have figure out what you believe is accurate and what you believe is not accurate.

J: Absolutely.

LRC: The other piece I would say—and then we'll close for the day—is I love this therapeutic mom piece. It's something that you're working on, Julie, and you'll know when you're ready to be a therapeutic mom.

J: Yeah.

LRC: Which is okay. And I really appreciate you're coming in today. I know how busy you are and so thank you so very much, Julie.

J: Thank you.

LRC: And I will see you in class tomorrow.

J: Tomorrow.

LRC: Thanks, Julie. I appreciate it a lot. Take care.

Summary

As stated earlier, theoretical specific or discipline specific supervision can be rich with supervision material. The strengths of this approach far outweigh the supervisor's fears of not being competent enough to help the supervisee. The supervisor may need to review counseling theories from the past, and if there is no solid knowledge base, then a referral or consultation may occur. If the supervisor is willing to stretch out of a familiar counseling zone, growth for both the supervisor and supervisee will occur. The supervisor needs to be cognizant, however, of the possible need for additional resources and models to round out the supervision needs.

Chapter Five Final Discussion Questions

1. Based on Julie's supervision question and her case presentation, how was the psychodynamic supervision model a wise choice? Find possible solutions in the chapter text.

_____

_____

_____

_____

_____

2. Think of a supervision moment when you as a supervisor or supervisee were observing a specific theoretical orientation skill. What would be the advantages of focusing on one theoretical orientation in supervision? Disadvantages? _____

_____

_____

_____

_____

_____

References

Bernard, J. M., & Goodyear, R. K. (1998). *Fundamentals of clinical supervision.* Needham Heights, MA: Allyn and Bacon.

Bowlby, J. (1988). *A secure base: Parent-child attachment and healthy human development.* New York: Basic Books.

Bradley, L. J., & Gould, L. J. (2001). Psychotherapy-based models of counselor supervision. In L. J. Bradley & N. Ladany (Eds.), *Counselor supervision: Principles, process and practice* (3rd ed.), Philadephia: Brunner Routledge.

Carta-Falsa, J., & Anderson, L. (2001). A model of clinical/counseling supervision. *The California Therapist, 13,* 47–51.

Corey, G. (2001). *Theory and practice of counseling and psychotherapy* (6th ed.). Pacific Grove: CA, Brooks/Cole.

Doehrman, M. (1976). Parallel processes in supervision and psychotherapy. *Bulletin of the Menninger Clinic, 40,* 3–104.

Ellis, A. (1989). Thoughts on supervising counselors and therapists. *Psychology: A Journal of Human Behavior, 26,* 3–5.

Frawley-O'Dea, M. G., & Sarnat, J. E. (2001). *The supervisory relationship: A contemporary psychodynamic approach.* New York: Guilford Press.

Goldstein, E. G. (2001). *Object relations and self psychology in social work practice.* New York: New York: Simon Schuster, Inc.

Hackney, H. L., & Goodyear, R. K. (1984). Carl Rogers' client-centered supervision. In R. F. Levant and J. M. Schlep (Eds.), *Client-centered therapy and the person-centered approach.* New York: Praeger.

Haynes, R., Corey, G., & Moulton, P. (2003). *Clinical supervision in the helping professions: A practical guide.* Pacific Grove, CA: Brooks/Cole.

Holloway, E. L. (1995). *Clinical supervision: A systems approach.* Thousand Oaks, CA: Sage.

Ladany, N., Friedlander, M. L., & Nelson, M. L. (2005). *Critical events in psychotherapy supervision: An interpersonal approach.* Washington, DC: American Psychological Association.

Lambers, E. (2000). Supervision in person-centered therapy: Facilitating congruence. In E. Mearns & B. Thorne (Eds.), *Person-centered therapy today: New frontiers in theory and practice* (pp. 196–211). London: Sage.

Liese, B. S., & Beck, J. S. (1997). Cognitive therapy supervision. In C. E. Watkins Jr. (Ed.), *Handbook of psychotherapy supervision* (pp. 114–133). New York: John Wiley & Sons.

Mikulincer, M., & Shaver, P. R. (2007). *Attachment in adulthood: Structure, dynamics and change.* New York: Guilford Press.

Morgan, M. M., & Sprenkle, D. H. (2007). Toward a common-factors approach to supervision. *Journal of Marital and Family Therapy, 33,* 1–17.

Patterson, C. H. (1997). Client-centered supervision. In C. E. Watkins Jr. (Ed.), *Handbook of psychotherapy supervision* (pp. 134–146). New York: John Wiley & Sons.

Pistole, M. C., & Fitch, J. C. (2008). Attachment theory in supervision: A critical incident experience. *Counselor Education & Supervision, 3,* 193–205.

Prouty, A. (2001). Experiencing feminist family therapy supervision. *Journal of Feminist Family Therapy, 12,* 171–203.

Prouty, A. M., Thomas, V., Johnson, S., & Long, J. K. (2001). Methods of feminist family therapy supervision. *Journal of Marital and Family Therapy, 27,* 85–97.

Rogers, C. R. (1961). *On becoming a person.* Boston: Houghton Mifflin.

Russell-Chapin, L. A. (2007). Supervision: An essential for professional counselor development. In J. Gregoire & C. M. Jungers (Eds.), *The counselor's companion: What every beginning counselor needs to know* (pp. 79–80). Mahwah, Nj: Lawrence Erlbaum.

Walsh, J. (2009). *Theories for direct social work practice.* Belmont, CA: Wadsworth/Cengage Learning.

White, M. B., & Russell, C. S. (1995). The essential elements of supervisory systems: A modified dephi study. *Journal of Marital and Family Therapy, 21,* 33–53.

Woods, P. J., & Ellis, A. (1996). Supervision in rational emotive behavior therapy. *Journal of Rational-Emotive & Cognitive Behavior Therapy, 14,* 135–152.

Social Role Supervision Models

Social Role Supervision Models

Social role supervision models tend to describe and organize what supervisors need to do rather than focus on a specific counseling theory (Holloway, 1995). These models acknowledge that, between them, the supervisor and supervisee have much wisdom and experience from professional role experiences, as well as a knowledge base and conceptualizations about counseling and the supervision process (Bernard & Goodyear, 2004; Casile, Gruber, & Rosenblatt, 2007). Three social role supervision models will be discussed.

Discussion Question 1

What are the benefits of emphasizing the roles that the supervisor might employ?

_____

_____

_____

_____

Bernard and Goodyear's Discrimination Supervision Model

The most widely known social role model is the discrimination supervision model. It has been extensively researched, and supporters of this type of supervision believe it is an inclusive approach to supervision, as it has its roots in technical eclecticism (Bernard & Goodyear, 1998). One of the main goals of the discrimination supervision model is to focus on the needs of the supervisee by being able to respond flexibly with any needed strategy, technique, and/or guidance.

It is situation specific, and supervisors emphasize two primary functions during each supervision session, that of the supervisor's role and focus. There are three roles that a supervisor takes based upon supervisee's needs: teacher, counselor, and consultant. Based on supervisory needs, the supervisor might put on the teacher's hat and directly instruct and demonstrate constructs and skills. The supervisor may need to be in the counselor's role to assist the supervisee in locating "blind spots" or perhaps in becoming aware of some personal countertransference issues. Finally, there may be times during supervision when what is required is a need for the supervisor to bounce back

OVERVIEW

Social role supervision models provide the benefit of identifying and emphasizing the varied roles and foci that supervisors need. These supervision models offer structure and interventions for both the supervisee and supervisor. They also assist the supervisory process by emphasizing the importance of interpersonal communication skills used by the supervisee.

GOALS

- Identify the varying roles and foci that supervisees need
- Understand when these models may be selected
- Identify fundamentals of the social role supervision models

and forth intervention ideas surrounding a client and become the supervisee's colleague and consultant (Russell-Chapin & Ivey, 2004; Russell-Chapin, 2007).

Each of these roles—teacher, counselor, and consultant—emphasizes three areas of focus for skill-building purposes: process, conceptualization, and personalization. Study and review the chart for the definition of each focal area.

Areas of Focus	
Role Focus	**Definition**
Process	Examines how you communicate with your client.
Conceptualization	Explores your intentions behind the chosen skill interventions
Personalization	Identifies mannerisms used to interact with clients such as body language, voice intonation

Basic Tenet

- Supervisees benefit from those supervisors who work from multiple theoretical orientations and focus on supervisee's needs by being able to respond flexibly with any needed strategy, technique, and/or guidance based upon the supervisor's role and focus.

When to Use

- When the supervisee is unaware of own experience with clients, the discrimination supervision model assists in expanding counseling knowledge base.

Supervisor's Roles and Behaviors

- The supervisor responds flexibly with needed role of teacher, counselor, and/or consultant guidance
- The supervisor selects the necessary focus.

Supervisor's Emphasis and Goals

- Emphasize two primary functions during each supervision session, that of the supervisor's role and focus.
- Three supervisor roles selected based upon supervisee needs are teacher, counselor and consultant.
- Each of these roles has three areas of focus for skill-building purposes.
- The three areas of focus are process, conceptualization and personalization.

Supervisee Growth Areas

- The supervisee will become more aware of personal areas needing improvement through interpersonal communications, the reasons behind counseling skill selection, and mannerisms.

Limitations

- There is limited empirical evidence testing the efficacy of the social role models (Holloway, 1992; Morgan & Sprenkle, 2007). This model may not be inclusive enough to meet all of the supervisee's needs.

Discussion Questions 2

1. How does the discrimination supervision model help the supervisee and supervisor discriminate among the roles, foci, and responses needed? _____

_____

_____

_____

_____

2. When using the discrimination supervision model, which of the foci would be most helpful to you as a supervisor and as a supervisee? _____

_____

_____

_____

_____

3. Which role would be the most difficult for you as a supervisor? _____

_____

_____

_____

_____

_____

Holloway's Social Role Supervision Model

Holloway (1995) created a similar model to the original discrimination model (Bernard, 1979) but added additional depth and complexity to the social role configuration by offering five supervisory functions, five tasks, and four general contextual factors (Morgan & Sprenkle, 2007). Holloway's 5 × 5 grid creates a process matrix for supervisors to determine the effectiveness of the selected tasks, functions, and methods (Morgan & Sprenkle, 2007).

The five functions and tasks interact with the four factors. The five functions are (1) monitor and evaluate, (2) instruct and advise, (3) model, (4) consult, and (5) support and share. The functions fall on a continuum of most structure and direction to less structure and more consultation. Lanning and Freeman (1994) added to this model another fundamental function that all supervisors need to address and model. Lanning (1986) believes the function of understanding and practicing professional and ethical behaviors is a must.

Basic Tenet

■ The Holloway social role supervision model believes in the importance of roles and foci but adds the additional supervisory functions, tasks, and contextual factors.

When to Use

- Use this supervision model when additional structure and evaluation is required to determine the effectiveness of the supervisee and supervisor.

Supervisor's Roles and Behaviors

- The supervisor uses the 5 × 5 process grid to examine the supervisory functions, tasks, and roles.

Supervisor's Emphasis and Goals

- The supervisor's main goal is to provide a comprehensive approach for conducting supervision using roles, foci, tasks, functions, and context.

Supervisee Growth Areas

- Through the evaluation system, the supervisee understands and works toward needed goals and liabilities. The supervisee moves from structured work and feedback to a collegial aspect as progress occurs.

Limitation

- The grid format assists in structuring the supervision process, but the grid can also be complex and intimidating to follow.

Discussion Questions 3

1. How do the additional five functions supplement this social role model? _____

_____

_____

_____

_____

_____

2. Why might adding the function of professional behaviors be important to the supervisory process? _____

_____

_____

_____

_____

_____

_____

Hawkins and Shohet's Social Role Supervision Model

Another major social role model of supervision is the six-foci approach of Hawkins and Shohet (2000). The six categories are interwoven into the two systems at work in supervision: the therapy and supervision systems. The six foci are (1) reflection on the content of the therapy session, (2) exploration of the strategies and interventions the counselor uses, (3) exploration of the therapy process and relationship, (4) focus on the counselor's countertransference, (5) focus on here-and-now process as a mirror or parallel of the there-and-then, and (6) focus on the supervisor's countertransference. These six foci are worked through within the contexts of counseling and supervision.

Basic Tenet

- In Hawkins and Shohet's social role supervision model, the main tenet emphasizes six foci and two systems.

When to Use

- Use this model when there is a belief that countertransference issues for both the supervisee and supervisor exist in counseling and supervision.

Supervisor's Roles and Behaviors

- Within the structure of foci and systems, the supervisor is an active director in the supervisory process.

Supervisor's Emphasis and Goals

- The major goal is to strategically and comprehensively maneuver through the six foci and the counseling and supervision systems.

Supervisee's Growth Areas

- The supervisee explores all aspects of the counseling process from content to parallel process.

Limitations

- This approach is comprehensive and time-consuming.

Discussion Question 4

In this social role supervision model, there are six foci to consider. In your mind, which foci might be more essential to the supervisory process? Are they equally important? Explain.

_____

_____

_____

As the reader begins to assimilate all the social role supervision models, again look for similarities and differences. This is the supervisor's and supervisee's opportunity to develop a unique and individualized model that works for the supervisory team.

DVD Supervisory Question

The supervision question that was offered to Lori assisted her in determining the best supervision model. Here is Kevin's question: "My client has switched coping mechanisms from cutting to tattooing. Now she wants even healthier coping strategies. How can I assist her in moving in that direction?"

Supervision and the Case of Kevin

Kevin's supervision question helped Lori key in on Kevin's supervision needs. First Lori selected the foci and role to use to accomplish the needed supervision goal and answer Kevin's supervision question. She chose to focus on Kevin's basic intervention skills by being in the role of teacher and counselor. Lori tried to teach new skills and understand Kevin's effect on the client.

The elegance of discrimination supervision is that as Lori continues to supervise Kevin, the foci and roles will change across sessions and within sessions (Bernard & Goodyear, 1998).

DVD Transcripts from the Case of Kevin

LRC = Dr. Lori Russell-Chapin
K = Kevin

LRC: Kevin, thank you so very much for joining me today. I know how busy you are, changing new jobs in the middle of all of this. I thought the best thing to do is start out by having you introduce yourself. Tell me a little bit about you. Maybe where you're headed in your profession, professional life, and then we'll focus on supervision.

K: Okay. Sounds great. I really appreciate this opportunity to speak with you as well. My name is Kevin McClure. I am a master's level therapist, also a licensed professional counselor with the state of Illinois.

LRC: That's exciting, Kevin. Very exciting. So you are headed on this second tier of counselor licensure in the state of Illinois, which is the Licensed Clinical Professional Counselor?

K: Correct. I'm finishing my hours over the next course of several months, and then I'll step forward in the fall.

LRC: So, Kevin, where do you—I mean, you're not just a brand-new counselor—where do you see supervision in your life?

K: Supervision for me right now is more about accountability, and building and honing my skills as a therapist for utilizing with my client. Really, not just the ones I don't know what to do with or I get lost in therapy with them. They really constantly challenge me to grow and continue to push myself as a therapist as well as my clients in their therapy.

LRC: So you can see it, again, playing several roles.

K: Absolutely.

LRC: To keep you on the cutting edge but to also provide that accountability piece. Right?

K: Absolutely.

LRC: Well, Kevin, tell me about the client you are bringing me today.

K: Today we are going to talk about a client—we'll call her Pat.

LRC: Okay.

K: A 45-year-old female Caucasian. Has some schooling. Spent some time working at an animal care clinic. She came to me about 2 years ago, actually during my internship. Really, the presenting problem was a general anxiety disorder. Specifically, social relationships. As we've done therapy, it really helped Pat to broaden her coping skills. We've done some assessments and found out that she scores pretty significantly on the borderline personality disorder axis as well.

LRC: What were you testing? What kind of test were you using?

K: We used the Coolidge Assessment Battery, which gives a wide range of the personality disorders, and mostly where she really scored clinically significant was the borderline personality disorder and anxiety disorders overall. So those really play a part. She is a lot more stable than she was, primarily because we got her in with a good psychiatrist who is doing some good med management with her but also a lot of psychotherapy to help her deal with issues, the trauma she dealt with as a child growing up.

LRC: Okay. Based upon that then, Kevin—I always like to put this back on you—what is your supervision question for today?

K: The thing I was thinking about most today—and I would really like your input—is throughout the course of therapy Pat has had a tendency to be a self-mutilator and cuts herself to relieve tension or anxiety or fear even. And recently, in the past 6 to 8 months, she has transitioned from cutting—self-mutilation—to tattooing. Which is—of course, is the same, but it's more socially acceptable. Recently, most recently, she is not sure tattooing is right for her as well. So, I see kind of this transition to a more and more healthy coping, and I'm wondering what should I look for next or where should I be helping her guide her in a more healthy helping?

LRC: Healthy direction. I mean, it's almost like she is changing addictions, sort of, but you're saying, "I would like her to get to a point where she can cope in a very constructive way."

K: Absolutely.

LRC: Okay. That sounds like a great place to focus. Let's do diagnosis on all five axes if you would, Kevin. If you've got your paper, please feel free to look at it.

K: Okay.

LRC: Go ahead and tell me. On Axis I again, presenting problems would be?

K: Presenting problem was 300.08 generalized anxiety disorder. That was the central core of why we started therapy. So then on Axis II, I diagnosed her with borderline personality disorder after getting the results back and sitting with an evaluation from a PhD. Axis III, medical concerns—most recently she found out she is middle of the transition of menopause. So I had menopausal transition there.

LRC: I think that could affect Axis I. I mean, I do think—we talk about even your supervisory question, which is coping strategies. I think all those things do work together.

K: Absolutely. And that's been huge; just putting a label on her hormonal and emotional ups and downs has been really good for her to say, "Oh, I'm not crazy. This is more biological." So just finding that out has really helped her get a sense of stability in herself as well. Axis IV, there are a lot of adjustment issues but mostly some parent–child relationship dysfunction going on there. That's long term, based upon her perception of abuse and the actual abuse that did occur.

LRC: Is that something that affects your main goal with her right now?

K: Her parents—although she lives at her parents' house and is custodian of the house while they are gone, they live primarily in Florida and she has limited contact with them. She is not dependent upon them anymore because she is now on half disability with the state, and is looking for a part-time job. We're helping job coach her as well for a part-time job. On the fifth Axis I have a current status or GAF score of 65. When she came to me, she was probably low 40s. She was significantly impaired.

LRC: Major improvement.

K: Major improvement over the past 2, 2½ half years.

LRC: Great. So again, the supervisor question we're trying to focus on is "How do I help her go into an even more healthy direction for coping?" And based upon that, Kevin, I'm trying to sit here and think about which supervisory model might be best, and I think what I would like to do—and I will share this with you—I think I would like to do something from a social role model of supervision. It's called the discrimination model, and I'll just share this with you, and then it will show up on the slides for somebody else who is watching. But the basic tenet would be that supervisees benefit from those supervisors who work kind of a theoretical model, so any theoretical orientation would work. But I'm also going to be trying to respond flexibly with any needs. Strategy, technique, or guidance—but I think the best time to use that would be when we're trying to have you be aware of maybe your own situations that might impede the counseling relationship. Again, Bernard's and Goodyear's discrimination model is a good example of these social role models. I have two things that I will try to do with you today, Kevin. One is that, as I said, I am going to try to respond flexibly with any needed role that you might need. So it could be I could put a counselor hat on. A teacher. Maybe a counselor. I don't suggest that I think that's a possibility, but—or maybe that of consultant again. And then, within each of these roles, Kevin, I would choose a particular foci or focus. So let me tell you a little bit about the focus. I could use either teacher, counselor, or consultant. Then the focus would be—we could process—in other words, we could process your communication style with Pat. That's one focus. We could talk about case conceptualization, which would really work on your intentions behind the skills you use. For example, if you're doing coaching, let's talk about the intention behind coaching and encouraging. Then the final stage is that of personalization, and this would be an interesting one too, Kevin, because it's just where I might identify certain mannerism that you use or vocal intonations that you might use. And you're smiling at me right now. So we can probably pick up on that as well.

K: Okay.

LRC: So we'll try if we can. I think I'm going to focus on this discrimination model with you.

K: Okay.

LRC: I guess the very first place though, Kevin, I need to start—and perhaps I'm using my teacher role, my teacher hat right now—but one of the things that you didn't share with me, but I know because I've had you in classes—but you also have a background of Native American heritage. Is that correct?

K: That's correct.

LRC: Tell me a little bit about that.

K: Well my mom is from the Pueblo Nation. The San Juan tribe in the southwest. She however, was adopted at a young age and I grew up very culturally educated from the Caucasian point of view. But over the last several years, my older brother and I have spent a lot of time investing in who are we are and trying to reconnect with that side of our family. We have yet to find them and locate them, but we are very fascinated by the spirituality, primarily, and the interaction of community that the Native Americans have. So that's just still part of my desire personally and professionally.

LRC: Sure.

K: It adds a lot.

LRC: I'll tell you why I went there, Kevin, is that I wonder with that background, we talk about diversity issues or multicultural issues. You're telling me you have a client who has had severe relationship kinds of issues and has struggled with men in general. I guess what I would want to know is how does she respond to you? You come from a very different background than she does, and to top it off, her Axis II diagnosis is that she's borderline. Do you know what I'm talking about, Kevin?

K: I think I know what you're asking.

LRC: There are so many different things going on, and I think we have to deal with that piece first. This multicultural issue first.

K: Okay. She has actually, through many years of recovery—she is 45 now—since probably 22 or 23 she has been seeking professional help, both psychiatric, inpatient/outpatient as well as psychological therapy, inpatient/outpatient. Her stories, her perception, is even abuse by professionals. She was misdiagnosed as dissociative identity disorder for years and went through just what she feels like is even trauma by the hands of professionals. So when she came to me and was assigned to me in the group practice—

LRC: As an intern, no less?

K: As an intern, no less—I was very nervous given her history that she was coming from. But what she wanted was a fresh start. She wanted kind of a new person that didn't have all the psychobabble—and all the things that would just relate to her. I think that is primarily what has really helped the therapeutic relationship between the two of us, because I treat her not just as a wounded person, but as a person. Not my patient, but as a person, and I think that does come from my spirituality and just my native American culture to relate to people as people.

LRC: And I guess that's what I want to get out of the way, Kevin. Have you specifically said to Pat, "Pat, you know, I might relate to you a little differently than other people because of who I am as just a person. It really doesn't have anything to do with Native American, but it's just who I am as a person, but I also have some Native American heritage and I really believe and I'm searching in that direction myself." Have you directly responded to Pat that way?

K: You know, I haven't really been that vulnerable with her because most of our sessions either really focus with anxiety-related issues or we do get into somewhat—she has really latched onto my compassion and how I really empathize with her and coach her and encourage her all the time because of her Axis II diagnosis. So we have spent—at least in the last six months of stability—spent a lot of time helping her differentiate the styles of relationships. Not just mine. And I haven't been that vulnerable about speaking about me, but we have talked about "Well, this might be this kind of relationship or that might be that kind of relationship, so don't expect all relationships to be the same. And don't expect everyone to always have the same kind of interaction with you." That's been kind of a growing-up process for her; because of her abuse and her trauma, she kind of missed out on the developmental years.

LRC: Absolutely.

K: As an adolescent and young adult.

LRC: Kevin, what I'm trying to get you to think about, though, is that—and these are the foci of this discrimination model as I have kind of been teaching—this piece

I want you to think about: you. And I recognize this as I've had you in class, you're a very intense and—you used the word beautifully—compassionate individual. And yet I think for someone that is borderline, I think you have to go very slowly with her, and I'm just suggesting that maybe, as she is becoming more comfortable with you, to address that piece of "I'm culturally different as well." Because, I think, one of the things we've learned through research on diversity is that we need to address our differences. It doesn't really mean too much, but we need to address them. And I think she even understands you as a male, as a caring, compassionate person, as someone who has a different heritage than she. Does that part make sense at all?

κ: It does make sense quite a bit. I think sometimes I get lost in not recognizing it and what I portray because I was raised from the Caucasian perspective. Cultural perspective.

LRC: Sure.

κ: So there's not always—a lot of times I think it doesn't react with me, so I appreciate you helping me remind me of that.

LRC: And I love that, Kevin, because it may not have anything to do with you. It just may have something to do with someone else who's saying, "Hmm. How come Kevin is so intense? How come he always looks me in the eye? I don't know if I want him to look me in the eye." And that could be Kevin—just you, Kevin—but that's that piece that I want you to consider.

κ: Okay.

LRC: Now, let's move on. Got that piece out of the way. I don't know if you believe this—and now I am kind of focusing from a consultant point of view.

κ: Okay.

LRC: But I sort of believe that when I get someone who has strong borderline personalities that it trumps everything that I do with them in therapy. Do you believe that or not?

κ: Well, I've definitely had weeks, even months, of "attempted therapy" with Pat that I really felt like we were just going around and around and around and around in circles. There would be times where, you know, I was "God" to her and she couldn't do anything without asking me. Or she would call and leave 15 hateful messages on my voicemail. I mean, it really went back and forth so quickly, and that started to change when I kind of confronted her. Not just compassionate, but with some boundaries. And put some boundaries in place for her. Not just from a—I want to say parental role with her—but even just in the therapeutic role, just to say, "This is not acceptable. This is not acceptable to treat me like this. I don't want to be your God but I'm not going to be your doormat either." I think that—she cried in that session, she was very upset with me, and it took about a week and a half to call me back to arrange the next session, but when she did, she said nobody had ever helped her see her own behavior.

LRC: Wow. That's the beauty, I think, Kevin, of providing structure, and I'm kind of in that teacher role again though, but I don't know if you've read the material on dialectical behavior therapy. Do you have that?

κ: I've read some of it. I haven't been trained in it yet.

LRC: I have several people who have, I'd say, severe borderline tendencies and even personality disorder, and I've gone so far to do the training, as well as there is a powerful book out. There's a workbook for your client, and I've gone through it because I think what she needs—it sounds like what Pat needs is such structure, Kevin. We have a homework assignment, we work on it, and we bring it back to the next session all the way through, because it's really teaching her how to relate and use emotions because she doesn't have those skills. That became very clear when you were talking. I want to just maybe throw that out to you to get into some of the workbook material on the dialectical behavior therapy.

ᴋ: Absolutely.

ʟʀᴄ: That kind of brings me back to your supervision question of "How do I help her go back to healthier skills?" Part of it is, I think, you're saying she's beginning to trust you.

ᴋ: Uh-huh.

ʟʀᴄ: And so she herself, in conjunction with you and other support systems, is moving from actually physically cutting herself to more socially accepted tattooing pieces. Talk to me a little bit about the tattoos. Tell me more about her tattoos. Do you know?

ᴋ: Well, she has a variety of them, and they've kind of marked different transition points, as I see them, related to her therapy and her overall stability. She was very afraid to get any tattoos at the very beginning, the beginning of her tattooing phase as I call it, because the family was not accepting of both. Accepting of it at all. She started with a little angel on the back of her shoulder as a representation of feeling as if somebody would always be with her.

ʟʀᴄ: Watching over her?

ᴋ: Watching over her. She's—at certain points, she has labeled different "personalities." At one point, she was diagnosed with dissociative identity, so there's one that has always stayed with her as kind of the father figure. The good father figure that she never knew. She named him Mike and she actually had a cartoon of him made and put way back in here. Kind of, as I see it, symbolic, to support her. Her whole inner structure. Her spine and everything.

ʟʀᴄ: The foundation piece.

ᴋ: The foundation piece. She had chains tattooed around her ankles, and most recently, I think, the last one that she had—she had a huge phoenix tattooed right here on her upper chest because she really felt like she had moved forward and had rebirthed beyond this horrible, traumatic victim. And really seeing herself as a survivor and someone who wants to do something with herself and help other people.

ʟʀᴄ: That's lovely, isn't it?

ᴋ: It is. Symbolically it's very incredible and that's why I never judged her and I never told her it was a bad thing. I just told her that she'd get a variety of responses. Some people would accept them and some people wouldn't and that it would be up to her to decide whether, really, this is what she wanted.

ʟʀᴄ: Well, Kevin, I want to go back to your supervisor question to make sure we get it answered today. I find that so interesting because it feels like every time she had a tattoo, it helped in this piece where she is growing. The phoenix piece, kind of. I love the idea of the angel on her shoulder. I like the idea of having the foundation in the back. The phoenix is sort of, "I'm coming out. I'm becoming a person." But she's now saying, "Do I have to physically hurt myself?"—although I have never had a tattoo, but I'm a big baby and so I think they're going to hurt.

ᴋ: She tells me it does hurt.

ʟʀᴄ: Okay. So, it seems to me it might hurt a little bit. Are there other ways she can cope and express herself without hurting herself? I'm going to throw back. I'm going to go back to this teaching piece again and maybe move into the conceptualization piece. I'm wondering, she sounds bright.

ᴋ: She's very bright.

ʟʀᴄ: I'm wondering if you might want to explore the union theoretic orientation with her, because in the union phase you get into masculine and feminine energies. You get into the feminine energies, which could be that receptive angel on her back. Masculine energies could be Mike, you know, on the foundation of her spine. And teach her things about the shadow and move into the things we repress into our shadow. And by doing that—and we can talk a lot more about this at another time—by doing that, I think what would happen, Kevin, it gets her to think about something outside of herself. It's not physical pain, but it gives her resources to deal with those issues.

K: Yeah.

LRC: So I'm wondering if you went down the union path with her, it might be really helpful.

K: I think that's a wonderful idea just from the standpoint that Pat responds very well to spirituality concepts and different things that are—and that's why I say she is very bright because she can think beyond the box. Beyond just logic. She can go ahead and think about metaphors and really understand them. So, I think that would be a good approach.

LRC: So then if we continue with the spirituality piece, though, Kevin, then once again it's even giving her resources within herself. Like masculine and feminine. Animus/anima kind of things—but then it's that spirituality piece, which is something outside of myself that I can access as a resource as well. I think that would be really helpful too. We can talk about that more, I think, at another supervision session. Kevin, let's do this. I'd kind of like to put some closing on this, and you can answer the question: What did we talk about today in supervision that you can take with you when you see Pat again? And before I do that, I've got to ask you this: I want to make sure we—you—had consent to tell us about Pat today. Is that correct?

K: Absolutely.

LRC: Written and verbal?

K: Verbal and written consent.

LRC: So I brought that piece. I just wanted to throw it in. Answer the supervision the question. I'm looking for outcome, Kevin. What will you take with you?

K: Well, I think the first thing that strikes me when you ask me that question is a reminder that I present myself differently than what most people might expect. So there are certain times in therapy that it's good just to bring that right to the forefront and acknowledge it.

LRC: Absolutely.

K: And just talk about it and allow people to be just more aware of that interaction and why that might be because of me or my heritage or a lot of different things that combine in that.

LRC: It's that immediacy piece though.

K: Exactly.

LRC: And Kevin, they may not think differently, but you might as well get it out in the open. Does that part make sense?

K: True. Absolutely. And the second piece is I like your suggested approach of doing more of the union style to help her build her external resources versus always feeling that she needs that internal kind, and then—

LRC: Kind of pain.

K: Then the physical pain. Right. And so trying to help her focus on the external resources so that she can continue to develop, to help with her transition.

LRC: I think both of those might work, and we'll keep talking more about Pat at another session. I guess what I wanted to talk about as we end today with the discrimination model, the reason I chose that for you, Kevin, is that it seems to me that I moved from teacher—I mean, I did a little of all of them; I did teacher, counselor, consultant. And then I looped into the different roles. I think we hit a lot of them. The process. Conceptualization. Personalization. And they are all kind of woven together, and you're saying you felt it was something you could actually use to work with Pat.

K: Well, you know, to me this model—I didn't really grasp when we were doing each one of those, but it did really happen, and I walk away with a lot to think about my client. I think that it's—for me again, where supervision is in my life—is that I need to walk away from supervision having ideas and thoughts about my client and knowing where to go next in therapy with them.

LRC: Well, it's almost like that's what we expect from our clients, and sometimes it nice to get that for ourselves.

K: Absolutely.

LRC: Kevin, thank you so very much for working with me. Congratulations on your new job too. And I will see you again in supervision soon.

K: It was wonderful. Thank you.

LRC: Thank you, Kevin.

Summary

Social role models of supervision offer the supervisor and supervisee essential structure to supervision sessions. Having the supervisor select the needed role and foci assists the supervisee in learning new skills, conceptual themes, and unknown factors inhibiting the counseling and supervision process.

Chapter Six Final Discussion Questions

1. Based on Kevin's supervision question and his case presentation, how was the supervisor successful in addressing the supervisee's specific needs? _____

_____

_____

_____

_____

_____

2. What are some of the advantages and disadvantages of selecting the discrimination supervision model for this supervisee. _____

_____

_____

_____

_____

_____

3. As a supervisor, what role and specific focus would you feel comfortable displaying with each of your supervisees? _____

_____

_____

_____

_____

4. Which roles and specific foci would be difficult for you? _____

_____

_____

_____

_____

References

Bernard, J. M. (1979). Supervisory training: A discrimination model. *Counselor Education and Supervision, 18,* 60–68.

Bernard, J. M., & Goodyear, R. K. (1998). *Fundamentals of clinical supervision.* Needham Heights, MA: Allyn and Bacon.

Bernard, J. M., & Goodyear, R. K. (2004). *Fundamentals of clinical supervision* (3rd ed.). Boston: Pearson/Allyn & Bacon.

Casile, W. J., Gruber, E. A., & Rosenblatt, S. N. (2007). Collaborative supervision for the novice supervisor. In J. Gregoire & C. Jungers (Eds.). *The counselor's companion: What every beginning counselor needs to know* (pp. 93–94). Mahwah, NJ: Lawrence Erlbaum.

Hawkins, P., & Shohet, R. (2000). *Supervision in the helping professions* (2nd ed.). Philadelphia: Open University Press.

Holloway, E. L. (1992). Supervision: A way of teaching and learning. In S. D. Brown & R. W. Lent (Eds.), *Handbook of counseling psychology* (2nd ed., pp. 177–214). New York: John Wiley & Sons.

Holloway, E. L. (1995). *Clinical supervision: A systems approach.* Thousand Oaks, CA: Sage.

Lanning, W. (1986). Development of a supervisor emphasis rating form. *Counselor Education and Supervision, 25,* 191–196.

Lanning, W., & Freeman, B. (1994). The supervisor emphasis rating form-revised: Counselor which roles and specific focus would be difficult for you? *Education and Supervision, 33,* 254–304.

Morgan, M. M., & Sprenkle, D. H. (2007). Toward a common-factors approach to supervision. *Journal of Marital and Family Therapy, 33,* 1–17.

Russell-Chapin, L. A. (2007). Supervision: An essential for professional counselor development. In J. Gregoire & Jungers (Eds.), *The counselor's companion: What every beginning counselor needs to know* (pp. 79–80). Mahwah, NJ: Lawrence Erlbaum.

Russell-Chapin, L. A., & Ivey, A. E. (2004). *Your supervised practicum and internship: Field resources for turning theory into practice.* Pacific Grove, CA: Brooks/Cole.

Integrated Models
of Supervision

Integrated Model of Supervision

Often when helping professionals are asked about their theoretical orientation, many clinicians will state they are eclectic in their views. To assist those who favor eclecticism, integrated models of supervision were designed for those who work from multiple theoretical orientations. Two approaches toward developing an integrated model are technical eclecticism and theoretical integration. Technical eclecticism takes techniques and interventions from many different theoretical orientations and uses them as needed without necessarily believing in a specific orientation. Theoretical integration, on the other hand, blends theoretical constructs and techniques from different theories to create a different and possibly better outcome for clients (Haynes, Corey, & Moulton, 2003; Norcross & Halgin, 1997).

Stoltenberg (2008) suggests there are three broad categories of supervision models: process-based, psychotherapy-based, and competency-based approaches. As discussed in previous chapters, process-based models focus on roles and tasks such as social role models, psychotherapy-based models emphasize specific counseling disciplines such as psychodynamic, and competency-based models highlight needed skills and best practice behaviors. The microcounseling supervision model discussed in the next section is an example of an integrated and competency-based approach to supervision.

Discussion Question 1

What could be advantages of conducting supervision using supervision models that are eclectic, integrated, and atheoretical? _____

_____

_____

_____

_____

Microcounseling Supervision Model

The microcounseling supervision model (MSM) falls into the category of integrated and competency-based supervision, as it is our belief that MSM successfully combines and uses many of the skills from a variety of theories and supervision models by

OVERVIEW

Integrated models of supervision tend to be atheoretical and use concepts from other counseling theories that are needed by supervisees. There are many ways that a supervisor and supervisee can formulate an integrated theory. Understanding the definition of integration and eclecticism is essential however. In this chapter, the integrated model of microcounseling supervision offers a standardized approach to supervision providing the supervisee strengths and areas for improvement. Follow along using the chapter transcription for a demonstration of the integrated microcounseling supervision model.

GOALS

- Understand the tenets behind integrated models of supervision
- Understand the differences between technical eclecticism and theoretical integration
- See how microcounseling supervision can be used with all supervision models

reviewing basic interviewing skills that are used in most theoretical orientations and counseling interviews (Russell-Chapin & Ivey, 2004b; Russell-Chapin, 2007). MSM combines both technical eclecticism and theoretical integration to create a supervision model that almost all counseling theories can use.

The beauty of MSM is that it teaches the supervisee and supervisor a natural method for reviewing counseling tapes and offering feedback, regardless of theoretical orientation. The microcounseling supervision model is a standardized approach assisting the supervisee in reviewing, offering feedback, teaching, and evaluating microcounseling skills. Lambert and Ogles (1997) described microcounseling skills as an approach that facilitates the general purposes of psychotherapy, no matter what the theoretical orientation. The effectiveness of microcounseling skills training has been researched for decades (Miller, Morrill, & Uhlemann, 1970; Scissons, 1993). In 1989, Baker and Daniels analyzed 81 studies on microcounseling skills training. Their finding concluded that microcounseling skills training surpassed both the no-training and attention-placebo-control comparisons. Daniels (2002) has followed microcounseling research for many years and now has identified over 450 data-based studies on the model.

Russell-Chapin and Sherman (2000) found, even with the effectiveness of the microcounseling approach, little consistency in the strategies used to actually measure and evaluate counseling students' skills and videotapes. Russell-Chapin and Sherman (2000) stated, "The need for quantifying counselor skills becomes increasingly important as the counseling profession continues to develop and refine standards for counselor competence" (p. 116).

The Counseling Interview Rating Form (CIRF) was designed in response to that very need to accurately and effectively supervise students' counseling videotapes and live supervision sessions (Russell-Chapin & Sherman, 2000). The CIRF has a variety of functions, but it's mostly used as a method of providing positive and corrective feedback for supervisee counseling tapes. For additional information about the construction, reliability, and validity of the CIRF, refer to Russell-Chapin and Sherman (2000).

The microcounseling supervision model (MSM) provides a vocabulary guide, a framework for constant examination of individual counseling style, and a method for offering feedback (Russell-Chapin & Ivey, 2004a). In beginning skills classes, students are encouraged to give others feedback. Usually the comments are very positive: "You were great," or "I liked the way you paraphrased." During supervision, though, more than positive feedback must be given. If constructive feedback is not provided to students during supervision, progress will be stagnant and perhaps nonexistent. This model offers a way for the supervisor and supervisee to learn to give constructive feedback incorporating strengths and areas for improvements by following the format of the Counseling Interview Rating Form (CIRF). This instrument can be utilized for qualitative and quantitative feedback for counseling interviews.

Discussion Question 2

Having a standardized approach to supervision has several benefits. Name two benefits that would meet your supervision needs. _____

_____

_____

_____

_____

The Counseling Interview Rating Form (CIRF)

A major component of microcounseling supervision is the Counseling Interview Rating Form (CIRF). The CIRF was originally developed for a counselor education program, but it has been used in both educational and clinical settings. The CIRF is the structured underpinnings of microcounseling supervision, as it provides a format for evaluating the five stages of the counseling interview as described by Ivey and Ivey (2003) and the microcounseling skills used in the counseling interview.

The CIRF was created by including the essential listening and influencing skills taught in many helping professional programs. Two categories of skills are included: (a) listening and influencing skills and (b) counseling interview stages. The CIRF is divided into six sections that correspond to the five stages of a counseling interview, plus one additional section on Professionalism. The vocabulary used for the five stages of the interview are (a) Opening, (b) Exploration, (c) Action, (d) Problem-Solving, and (e) Closing sections. Listed within each section are skills or tasks that are seen in that stage of the interview. The Opening section, for example, includes the specific criteria of greeting, role definition, administrative tasks, and beginning. A blank CIRF is included in Appendix C.

Discussion Question 3

After looking over the CIRF in Appendix C, jot down any questions about the form. Discuss in your supervisory team. When will the CIRF be most effective for you to use? _____

_____

_____

_____

Scoring the CIRF

While watching a videotape or participating in a live counseling supervision session, a supervisor or supervisory team uses the CIRF to tally the number of times a certain skill is used. If the skill is demonstrated five different times, a frequency mark would be entered each time. Values are assigned after the counseling session to indicate the level of mastery achieved for each skill, and ratings of 1, 2, or 3 for each of the 43 listed skills are given for those skills observed.

Ivey and Ivey (2003) describe mastery as using the skills with intention, with an observable, desired effect on the client. A score of 1 is offered if the counselor used that skill with little or no effect on the client; a score of 2 says the counselor used the skill with mastery and intention; and a score of 3 indicates the counselor was demonstrating and teaching a new skill or concept to the client. A score of 3 is used sparingly.

The CIRF includes space for comments next to each skill, so any reviewer can make notes or write the counselor's actual statements while viewing the tape. These comments are extremely important to the supervisory session, as they can offer the counselor true examples of skills and processes used during the interview. The last page of the CIRF consists of space for providing written feedback on the strengths and noting areas for improvement. During microcounseling supervision, all peer supervisors and the instructor will use the narrative space to provide constructive feedback.

When the CIRF is used for quantifying counseling sessions into grades, the total values are tallied, with an A corresponding to 52 points and higher (i.e., at least 90% of the total points).

This cut-off score requires scoring in the mastery range on all the essential skills denoted by an "X" on the CIRF. Essential skills are those deemed necessary for an effective interview as determined by the CIRF authors and the microcounseling approach to training (Russell-Chapin & Sherman, 2000).

Uses of the CIRF

The CIRF is useful as an evaluative tool for supervisors and peers and for self-evaluation. By using this form as a central foundation to microcounseling supervision, you can approach supervision time with less vulnerability, as the environment to supervision is not threatening but validating. In addition to an evaluation tool, the CIRF is an excellent teaching tool. Use the CIRF to identify areas and skills frequently used and those skills not being used.

The Three Components of Microcounseling Supervision

The microcounseling supervision model has three major components: (1) reviewing skills with intention, (2) classifying skills with mastery, and (3) processing supervisory needs. Its tenets are based on microcounseling skills first reported by Ivey, Normington, Miller, Morrill, and Haase (1968), and all the skills correspond to the five stages of the counseling interview.

Reviewing Microcounseling Skills with Intention

The first component of the microcounseling supervision model is essential to the efficacy and efficiency of the remaining sections. Supervisees must review each of the basic interviewing skills and understand their intention. Once a supervisee is comfortable and secure with defining and reviewing the microcounseling skills, then the supervisor can assist the supervisee in rapidly entering into the second phase. It is critical that initially the supervisee takes the needed time to ensure that each individual skill definition along with the underlying intention of that skill is understood. Intention is defined as choosing the best potential response from among the many possible options.

In the first MSM stage, the supervisee is not looking for the "right" solution and skill, but is selecting responses to adapt individual counseling style to meet the differing needs and culture of clients (Ivey & Ivey, 2003). With intentionality, supervisees can anticipate specific interviewing results if certain skills are used! For example, if a supervisee wants a client to continue expressing emotions, a basic reflection of feeling would be a wise skill to choose. A client laments, "Today was my little boy's first day of kindergarten!" The counselor's reflection of feeling is, "There must be many differing emotions going on inside. You could be sad, lonely, scared yet excited!" Review the first step of microcounseling supervision by practicing, defining, and reviewing all the microcounseling skills. A glossary of the 43 microcounseling skills with their intentionality is provided in Appendix D.

Discussion Question 4

Review the glossary of 43 microcounseling skills. Which of those skills need additional clarification? Discuss them with your supervisory team. _____

_____

_____

Classifying Skills with Mastery

The second stage of the MSM is Classifying Counseling Skills with Mastery. One of the easiest methods to begin the second stage is to have examples of someone else demonstrating the microcounseling skills and their uses. When your supervisee is comfortable, allow her to watch a videotape of her own, and classify the skills observed using the CIRF. The two of you could share your scores and classifications. Look for the areas of agreement and those areas that are missing.

Summarizing and Processing Supervisory Needs

The final stage of the microcounseling supervision model begins by summarizing and processing the demonstrated skills on the CIRF, as well as other important dimensions of the session. Using the Counseling Interview Rating Form (CIRF), begin summarizing skill usage with frequency tallies. Go through the transcript again and use a frequency tally for each of the counseling responses observed. At the end of the session or during each response, see which of the responses represent basic mastery and active mastery. Remember basic mastery is defined as being able to demonstrate the skill during the interview, and active mastery shows the supervisee producing specific and intentional results from the chosen counseling skill.

The final step is to compare the reader's rating with the authors'. In a regular classroom or a supervision session this final step will be discussing supervisee ratings with classmates and supervisors. Once the CIRF has been tallied by the members of the supervisory team, the narrative process for microcounseling supervision can begin. The student counselor will present the interview video and case presentation ahead of time and has been asked to formulate needed supervisory questions and concerns. These issues are addressed as a team in a round-robin fashion going over supervisory concerns, strengths, and areas of improvement. The very last question asked would be "What did you learn in supervision today that will assist you in more effectively working with this client?" Many of these comments may come from the Strengths and Area for Improvement area of the CIRF. The comments on these sections will help the supervisee immensely to progress forward (Russell-Chapin & Ivey, 2004).

Basic Tenet

- Supervisees benefit from a standardized, atheoretical approach assisting them in reviewing, offering feedback, and evaluating micro- and macrocounseling skills and the counseling interview.

When to Use

- When essential microskills are not effectively utilized, selecting the microcounseling supervision model is suggested.

Supervisor's Roles and Behaviors

- Use the Counselor Interview Rating Form (CIRF) as a mechanism for creating a reciprocal supervision process for offering constructive feedback.
- Choose from the three MSM components based upon supervisee's needs: Reviewing Skills with Intention, Classifying Skills with Mastery, and Processing Supervisory Needs.

Supervisor's Emphasis and Goals

- Assist the supervisee with clarifying and defining all micro- and macrocounseling skills.
- Identify and classify observed skills with intention using the CIRF.
- Process the strengths and liabilities of the counseling session answering the supervisory question.

Supervisee's Growth Areas

- The supervisee begins to better understand and classify all micro- and macrocounseling skills.
- The supervisee progresses to the mastery level of skill development.

Limitations

- The major limitation is that MSM is best utilized when there is a videotape or digital tape of a counseling session. In some settings obtaining a recording of a counseling session does not easily occur.

DVD Supervisory Questions

This supervisee's questions were twofold:

- Susan seems to be doing well in this stage of sobriety. Could you give some guidelines as to when to push and when to back off?
- Once I get to process-oriented material, what do I do?

The Supervision Case of Cate

Cate asked several supervision questions. After watching her videotape, it seemed she was missing several basic skills, so the integrated microcounseling supervision model made sense to use.

The cardinal rule of any integrative supervision is to customize supervision to meet the needs of the individual supervisee. In other words, "the 'how' of supervision should parallel the 'what' of supervision" (Norcross & Halgin, 1997, p. 210). Lori chose to demonstrate with Cate how and what could be accomplished by answering her supervision questions.

DVD Transcripts from the Case of Cate

LRC = Lori Russell Chapin
  C = Cate

> **LRC:** Thank you so much for joining me today in supervision. I really appreciate it. I know how busy you are with teaching and doing internships, so thanks for joining me today.
>
> **C:** Well, thank you for inviting me. I'm honored to be involved in this project.
>
> **LRC:** Well, I think it's been fun, Cate, so I really do appreciate your time. Why don't we first start off just having you introduce yourself a little bit, and then we'll move right into your case.
>
> **C:** Okay. My name is Cate Catherine Phiefer. I have a PhD in communications from the University of Wisconsin. I teach at Bradley.

LRC: Wisconsin?

C: Wisconsin. Wisconsin. Anyway, I teach at Bradley and I teach advertising and public relation courses, and I'm also getting a master's in counseling.

LRC: So you are a nontraditional student and you'll be changing career fields soon?

C: I probably will. In fact, I'm an extreme nontraditional student because I'm also a Buddhist. I've been a Dharma teacher for 5 years and have practiced medication for about 14.

LRC: So you bring to the counseling profession a lot of diversity, Cate?

C: I do. I do.

LRC: Right. Well, then let's go in. Let's talk a little about your supervision question. Maybe start with a telling me a little bit about your client, Cate.

C: Okay. Her name is Susan and she has gone through a rather intensive therapy process for substance abuse. Specifically, for pharmaceuticals, and she has just recently finished that program and is going through the adjustment of getting back into the world. Finding a new job and things like that as a sober person. So that's basically it. She has actually started a job right after we did our interview.

LRC: Wow.

C: So, yes. She's being moved into the real world again. There's a lot of transition there in her life.

LRC: Good. Let's do a couple of things. First of all, do we have Susan's consent to be showing the tape?

C: We do.

LRC: And doing supervision.

C: Yes, we do. We have both verbal and written.

LRC: Okay. Let's back up a little bit and talk about her diagnosis on all five axes. On Axis I, which would be the reason she came into treatment, it would be what?

C: It would be substance abuse.

LRC: Okay. And Axis II? Any personality disorder?

C: We didn't have tests for that, so that is deferred.

LRC: Deferred? Axis III would be her medical conditions. Any medical conditions that relate to her Axis I?

C: It's unknown at this time. Not that we know of.

LRC: So she's fortunate then.

C: She is fortunate that she hasn't ruined her health with this.

LRC: Axis IV would then be psychosocial stressors, Cate. Talk about those.

C: Well, right now, presently, she is going through quite an adjustment. She was going to the drug rehab center daily, and now she is on her own in her own apartment and finding a job. She had gone through all the legal things that sometimes pop in for abuse issues. So, right now, she is going back to what we consider a more normal life. She is normalizing.

LRC: Good. And so I remember—watching your tape too—one of the things I think was a concern of hers was the relationship with her husband.

C: Well, that's . . .

LRC: That happens.

C: Yeah. There has been a cycle of substance abuse for so long that now everything is changing. You know. Her habits are changing. Her life is changing. She not going to the old playground and being with the old playmates, as we say in the field.

LRC: Okay. How about Axis V? What would you give her as a Global Assessment Function score?

C: Well, she's functioning quite well. At the end of her treatment, she was actually teaching and a leader among her group. And so I think she is functioning at 75? Maybe a little higher than that?

LRC: Higher than that? So the prognosis for you is saying, "I think she is functioning well and probably she will do rather well."

C: That is the prognosis. Yes.

LRC: Even though the rate of recidivism is so high in substance abuse?

C: Yes. Yes. And she has a particular concern too, and we talked about it on the tape. She's a nurse, and access to these pharmaceuticals that she was addicted to had a high rate, so she needed to find a job in her field that wasn't going to be tempting or dangerous for her.

LRC: For her or for other people around her.

C: Exactly.

LRC: Well, Cate, so the supervision question again: What would be your supervision question? Or questions that we could focus on today on supervision?

C: Well, one of my questions is about somebody going through rehabilitation. How much do you push, because there's a certain—you know, honesty and confrontation within therapy, but also somebody who has gone through the difficulties of going through rehabilitation also needs cheerleading. I need to know what the balance is in that. And, you know: know when to hold them, know when to fold them. I'm also interested in—and this process we're going through with my internship or now my practicum and now my internship is, I want to go into more process-oriented counseling.

LRC: Uh-huh.

C: Because there's more cerebral—the CVT and things like that—but as a counselor I'm going to need a range of skills to be effective. So—

LRC: Excuse me, Cate, for interrupting what you're saying. So, what I like to know is—be able to dig a little deeper. Get away from the story and move into process a little bit more.

C: Exactly. And once I get there, what do I do?

LRC: Okay. All right. Well, you know, what I have been trying to demonstrate today is that there are different models based upon supervisee needs. As I listen to you, Cate, the model I'd like to demonstrate with you is the microcounseling supervision model. It's the one that you're very familiar with in class because we use it all the time.

C: Excellent.

LRC: When I bring out this form, most people kind of go, "Oh, I see that form again. Haven't seen it in quite a while." I'm going to bring out your form, which means that I have watched your tape and I have gone through it, actually. Look at all the skills that you are doing. And I think by doing that we can answer your two supervision questions. So, the first thing I think I want to do—just so the viewers, as they are watching, can understand. Microcounseling supervision is an example of an integrative model of supervision. It means it's atheoretical; it doesn't use any particular theoretical orientation.

C: Uh-huh.

LRC: And here's the basic tenet. The supervisees benefit from a standardized—there it is again—atheoretical approach. The system in reviewing, offering feedback, which is what you asked me for—and maybe you don't want to know it, Cate—but evaluating micro- and macrocounseling skills and also talking about the counseling interview itself.

c: Okay.

LRC: Again, I would use this specifically when trying to focus on particular skills—like you said: "How do I move from content to process?" I think that's probably a good selection for you. The example would be—this is a model that I created a long time ago, Cate, probably in 1999. It started to be published in 2004 and now it's in a textbook, and so I think it has a particular use when we are trying to focus on skills.

c: Uh-huh.

LRC: The roles and behaviors would be [the ones] that use this nasty Counseling Interview Rating Form that you use in class all the time. It's not nasty. We use that first and it helps us create this, I think, reciprocal feedback. You've done your own tape. You've seen it already. Now I've done it, so now we can kind of compare and contrast.

c: Excellent.

LRC: And then there are three components of microcounseling supervision. The first one is reviewing skills with intention.

c: Right.

LRC: The second one is classifying skills, and I'll talk about each of these. And then the last one is processing everything we've seen. So I think by doing that, again, we can answer your questions, Cate. Let's go through real quickly each one of those stages.

c: Okay.

LRC: The first one would be when I look at this skill, this Counseling Interview Rating Form, I have a feeling I know the answer, but as you look at any of these skills, Cate, which of these might you need some clarification on? Anything? Any skill?

c: Well, I think I need more material over here in this action phase. It seems a little sparse.

LRC: Okay.

c: And I see that there's a bit of a gap here in the problem solving.

LRC: One of the things that I noticed on your Counseling Interview Rating Form is that she said this is a good place to put some special techniques. So we can talk and clarify that too. It was interesting on your form, Cate, where I put process. It doesn't mean this is right or wrong, but where I put process, you were calling it a special technique.

c: Oh.

LRC: And I think it does overlap. I do think the skills overlap, but other than that you want to check out the voids in here—but are there any particular definitions that you need, Cate? That you can think of?

c: I would say that I would like to know what is a special technique and how do we implement alternatives?

LRC: Okay. Let's do that very quickly then. I think a definition of a special technique would be probably, Cate, if you chose to teach someone meditation. That's just an example. And that you kind of put on that teacher hat and you say, "I want to teach you specifically how to meditate," and maybe teach them how to breathe correctly. That would be an example of a special technique. The implementing alternative one, I think, is really important, and that's what I want to talk about today with you because it's like you get so far and then you stop. For example—and this will make sense in a little bit—you talk about her triggers. Her going back into the real world and are you exposing yourself to triggers? What are you doing with that? Then you even say, "Well what are you doing when you come across something that is a trigger for you?" And then you don't say to her—which is the answer to your next question, implementing alternatives—you don't say to her, "Okay. Let's have a plan so that the next time your get a trigger you'll know what to do." That would be the actual implementation.

c: Okay.

lrc: All right. So that's the first phase of microcounseling supervision where we go through these micro- and macroskills and say, "Are you clear on them?" The second stage is what you've already done, where you're classifying. Either you can watch someone else do this, Cate, or—you did it. You did counseling. You did it on videotape and then you started scoring your own form just like I did. What I thought was really interesting, again, is that most of the time we had—most of the time what I saw and observed, you saw and observed. But there were a couple of times where there were things that I didn't see. That doesn't mean they weren't there, and so we'll talk a little bit about that too.

c: Okay.

lrc: At this stage though, Cate, this is where, when we classify skills with intention, you were really starting to think about "Why did I do that?"

c: Yes.

lrc: That's that intention piece, and so on this particular form when you score something with intention, you are saying, "Not only did I do it with intention, but the outcome was effective. If the client did what I thought she would do—so when I paraphrase, I did it purposefully, and she said, 'Oh, she really wants me to talk more.'" That's the beauty, I think, of intention.

c: Okay.

lrc: And then the last part of this model, Cate, is when we process your supervisory needs. So I go through all this with you and then I come up with—on the back page there's strengths and weaknesses.

c: Okay.

lrc: And you always say to me, "Oh my gosh, there's more on the areas for improvements than there are the strengths." And I say, "No, no. That's not true. I just write really big on this one."

c: Well, that—and also it's a roadmap. It shows me the areas that I do know and it helps me sketch out those areas I'm trying to work on.

lrc: Okay. Well then let's go through this, Cate. I thought what was really interesting as I look through this is that every single one of these basic microcounseling skills you answered, and several times you answered them and you had a frequency tally of many of them. For example—I'm sure there were more—but there were like six or seven open-ended questions that you did. For example, "What kind of job would you want?" Those kind of things. I thought you did beautifully on the examples of reflection of feelings. Reflection of meaning. You're really getting those. I love that you can do those reflections of meaning. I didn't see—you said you did—I did not see you do some summarizations. Although when you did this form you said, "I did some."

c: Uh-huh.

lrc: Summarizations to me would be these wonderful paraphrases that you do to help you go into a new transition.

c: Okay.

lrc: It doesn't mean that I—they really could be there, Cate—I just didn't see them, so we might want to watch for that another time.

c: Okay.

lrc: So a lot of those basic microcounseling skills weren't there. You already observed—though I didn't see this implementation of alternatives. Which, I think then, moves you right into this next piece, where you said, "I see a bunch of voids." I didn't see a lot of the action phase, Cate. I saw genuinely good listening skills.

c: Uh-huh.

lrc: Reflection I saw. But I didn't see this piece here, which is action phase.

c: Uh-huh.

lrc: I saw some nice generalizations, and I felt you were very appropriate professionally and developmentally with her.

c: Thank you.

lrc: You're welcome. So let's move in—specifically into the last piece, which is the processing of your supervisor needs.

c: Okay.

lrc: Go ahead and reiterate the supervisory questions. One was about process.

c: One was about process and the other was about how much to push and how much to cheerlead and how to get that appropriate balance for the client at that time. Because I know sometimes we'll want to push the client more, and sometimes we'll want to cheerlead more, and sort of know when to do each of these.

lrc: Okay. Let me ask you the question first: Were you a leader and pusher today or were you more of the cheerleader in this tape?

c: I'd say in this tape I was more of the cheerleader. Actually, in the transition period she was exhibiting many actions and many thoughts that were really going to help her. She was going in a good direction and I wanted her to know that.

lrc: I thought she was functioning very autonomously on this, Cate. She had good insight. She'd ask the question and she'd say, "Well, I want to do this." She was well planned, so I can see why you were being more of a supporter. However, I felt that—this is the balance piece I'm trying to answer in your question—I felt you missed some opportunities, Cate.

c: Uh-huh.

lrc: I think that is what you're working on right now. How do I be a cheerleader and a confronter? Can you do both? And I think the answer is absolutely. You can do both.

c: Good.

lrc: And here are some of the missed opportunities. If you go back to your page, see if this makes any sense to you.

c: Uh-huh.

lrc: She says that she still struggles with trust. That her husband doesn't trust her yet with money. That a lot of family members don't trust her yet.

c: And that's a classic issue with people who are going from treatment back into their lives because they say addiction is cunning, baffling, and powerful.

lrc: That's good.

c: At the end, people will go to extremes to get their next fix.

lrc: And so, you know, she is saying, "I'm following this normal path. I can understand why people don't trust me." But what you said then was—which was nice and that was one of your strengths. I thought you did great verbal tracking. When she talked, you continued to track with her, Cate. I appreciated that. But rather than asking a question, which was, "What would you say the biggest issue you're struggling with trust is?" I would do some reflection. I would say because that is going to get you deeper into that process question too. Or that issue too. So I thought there were some missed opportunities with process and with trust.

c: Okay.

lrc: Let's just see if I can get there with you. For example—and I thought there was one point on the tape that was really nice, Cate, where she had finished her statement and you chose intentionally, I think, to be silent. But then you did this. You were silent and then—I know you remember this—then you went, "So?" And she goes, Susan goes, "So?" And then you both begin to laugh. I wonder if the missed opportunity, Cate, might not have been to say, "Susan, what . . ."—and you could still laugh, and I love the sense of humor you have, and we have talked about this, Cate. Though occasionally it gets you in trouble because it takes the heat off.

c: Yep.

lrc: Rather than staying focused and getting to the process. I thought this was a chance where you could have said, "Okay, Susan." She says, "What I need from other people sometimes is a small bit of acknowledgment. I want my husband to say, 'I think you're doing a pretty decent job.'" Which is always that external piece again.

c: Right.

lrc: I wondered if you could have said, "But you know, there must be a way you can acknowledge yourself, Susan."

c: So to give the internal locus of control?

lrc: Absolutely. Then we're dealing with that focus piece again. Get her back into herself. Not always saying, " I want something to validate me." I think that's one of her addiction problems in the beginning. She was always searching to make her okay.

c: Uh-huh.

lrc: Rather than focusing on there have to be ways you can acknowledge yourself.

c: Uh-huh. And this is just one of the examples that we talked about earlier. I get the swing, but I don't go all the way through.

lrc: Cate, I think that's it. Because you are really good at intentionally listening and reflecting.

c: Uh-huh.

lrc: And then it was kind of like, "Okay." It's like—you know, even though I think maybe you hit the ball. The ball actually hits the bat, but it's not going to go as far or as effectively because it's not hit with direction.

c: Uh-huh.

lrc: And so I guess I'm asking you to think about ways you can focus on her and say, "How, Susan, can you acknowledge yourself so that you're not always disappointed when other people don't recognize your progress or your big battles that you're winning?"

c: Uh-huh.

lrc: Does that part make sense?

c: It does make sense. Trust is such a basic need. It's such a big issue. It needs to be explored.

lrc: And that's that process piece, Cate. That's the supervisory question on process. Let me see if there are any others that I thought would be fun for process. Here's another one; here's a process piece. She was concerned about happiness, so I thought you could put on your teacher hat and talk about the three components of happiness. The most recent research on positive psychology is talking about this whole thing that there are three components. There's the pursuit of happiness. Pursuit of pleasure. There's the "What do we need from meaningfulness?" And also, how well does she engage? I think Susan has enough of an idea of who she is about pursuit of pleasure. Less addiction. I'm not talking about that kind of pleasure.

c: Right.

LRC: I think she has that piece.

c: Uh-huh.

LRC: I don't know if she knows yet the meaningfulness piece, Cate. What gives her meaning in her life?

c: Uh-huh.

LRC: Does she know that piece yet?

c: I would guess right now, no. There's so much transition that that's something she needs to be more grounded in.

LRC: And I think that's a process piece that you could hit on too. It goes back to that acknowledgment of self. The third component of happiness is that whole piece of engagement. "How do I actually connect with other people?"

c: Uh-huh.

LRC: And so we're getting her out of her story.

c: Uh-huh.

LRC: And we're moving her into understanding and process.

c: Okay.

LRC: So, I think that's one thing I would really like you to focus on. If I answer your second—or first or second supervision question, this piece about, "How do I be the cheerleader and the confronter at the same time?" I guess I'd go back to this, Cate. You said, "I think I'm probably more of the cheerleader in this tape."

c: Yes.

LRC: I'm asking you a purposely closed question. Do you have a good relationship with her? Do you have rapport with this woman?

c: Yes.

LRC: And you said it very emphatically. "Yes, I do."

c: Uh-huh.

LRC: Then you know if you've got rapport with someone that you can confront them.

c: Uh-huh.

LRC: So, Cate, if I'm Susan now, what do you want to say to me?

c: I would probably ask questions of exploring what's she doing to build trust? Or what's she doing to trust herself?

LRC: Oh, I like that one.

c: Uh-huh.

LRC: Okay. And so we'll explore those kind of things about trust, but talk to me a little bit more about—what I am trying to get you to think about is this engagement piece and this acknowledgement piece. Is there something that you would have to do to confront her? That's the piece that I want you to get. See, one of your big strengths, Cate, is that you're a great thinker. You're a wonderfully intellectual person, but I want you to deal with the feeling part of this. What do you want to say to Susan? Confront her. What's the discrepancy that I'm feeling?

c: Right now, nothing's coming to mind, but we're obviously going towards the feeling aspects.

LRC: We're going toward the feeling part. What are you afraid of for her, Cate?

c: What am I afraid of?

LRC: Not you personally. Well, I'd like to know that, but that's a whole other time.

c: No, but for her?

LRC: Yeah.

c: I would be afraid that by not feeling the trust that she craves, she would go for something else she craves.

LRC: Yeah.

c: That would be my largest concern.

LRC: That's what you need to ask her.

c: Uh-huh.

LRC: And what's really interesting about your supervision questions is that they are just so closely intertwined that they answer each other. If you confront her, you get into process.

c: Uh-huh.

LRC: Can you see that?

c: I see that.

LRC: That's what I want you to do. Now, let's go back though—it could be Freudian, I don't know—but let's go back to what are you afraid of, Cate, in doing that?

c: In doing that?

LRC: Yeah. What are you afraid of in not being her cheerleader but being a balance between cheerleader and confronter?

c: I would say that there would be a couple of things I'm afraid of. One of them would be that I am not being effective—

LRC: Okay.

c: —would be one thing, because something like confrontation you don't do lightly.

LRC: Uh-huh.

c: That's something you purposefully choose. You have to have intentions for it.

LRC: Well—and Cate, here's what I want to share with you though. But I think maybe I want you to recognize this, that there's an old counseling cliché that sometimes I just hate, but sometimes if you confront someone, you really do care about them. To confront someone doesn't mean that you have to be nasty to them. It's done in a caring way because you have trust and rapport with this woman.

c: Okay.

LRC: So you will be effective if you trust yourself enough to say, "I'm going to tell you what my big fear is for you." Because as soon as you do that, Cate, Susan will say, "Let me tell you what my big fear is."

c: Uh-huh. So you get to a deeper level for both of you.

LRC: Absolutely.

c: It's not that one's up here and one's down there.

LRC: And what will happen in counseling, Cate, is that both of you, the counselor and client, get to a deeper level.

c: Effective counseling that might help both.

LRC: I think much deeper effective counseling, and you eradicate your biggest fear by going there. That's what I think is so powerful.

C: Uh-huh.

LRC: So let's do this. I'm going to give you this. This is my form and then—

C: Thank you.

LRC: Oh, yes. I'm sure you're just dying to have that, Cate. But I guess what I'll have you do is take a look at everything. You can look at the inside and the outside. Look at the voids. Look at it and talk to me about it, and it doesn't mean that my view is correct, Cate, and talk to me about what we did in supervision that will help you work with Susan again.

C: Okay. I'd say we answered my questions—which is actually multilayered because there's the "Where do I go from here?" You know, the follow-through.

LRC: The hitting the bat and following through?

C: Right. And hitting her core issues because ultimately I think that would be the most helpful. There's an awful lot of psychoeducation material that appears in rehabilitation.

LRC: Uh-huh.

C: Drug rehab. She's gone through all that and so when we have one-on-one time— because most of the program I'm working in, most of the drug rehabilitation is in groups—you know, I want to use this time for its best purpose.

LRC: As effectively and efficiently as possible.

C: Right. Because we often don't have a lot of time.

LRC: Uh-huh.

C: So that is a big issue and, you know, I guess I'm looking to not only be effective but—I don't know—inspire her for more insights.

LRC: Uh-huh.

C: If I could pick the domino that keeps her exploring, I'd say that's the most effective I could be.

LRC: I think that that will happen. What I find interesting about this is that you are willing to practice what you talk about in supervision.

C: Uh-huh.

LRC: Then these skills will all be there.

C: They will.

LRC: There's implementation of alternatives. There'd be a special technique if you'd get into those trust issues. I can see you teaching her some of the spirituality issues that would be a powerful resource for her.

C: Trusting in your higher power.

LRC: Yes. I didn't see the focus thing, which you put right back on her when you said, "Come on, Susan. How can you acknowledge yourself rather than expecting your husband to do that?"

C: Uh-huh.

LRC: Then I see confrontation and so what that would do for me is—and this is the purpose of microcounseling supervision—I began it in the beginning to teach. I wanted to look at a whole counseling tape, and I want to be able to quantify a whole tape because I have to give you grades. Right?

C: Uh-huh.

LRC: But it turned out to be a quantitative and qualitative piece because now the qualitative piece is we get into these wonderful statements and issues that we talked about.

But as I quantified your tape—and I want you to think about this, and this is not easy to do—but if you had to give yourself a grade on this tape what would it be?

c: I'm a tough grader.

lrc: Okay.

c: I'd give myself probably a B.

lrc: Okay.

c: And the reason I would do that is I know I missed a big part of this.

lrc: Piece of it.

c: A big piece of this. I also know that I did many of the skills very well.

lrc: Absolutely.

c: I also feel that I haven't arrived yet, but I feel like I'm going in a good direction.

lrc: Cate, that's interesting because normally—I mean I can grade this quantitatively and qualitatively. Qualitatively, you did demonstrate a lot of the skills, and they were done with intentions and effectively. Quantitatively, I would give you a B+ on the tape. It wasn't that you missed a big piece. It was that process piece. It was that getting her out of content and moving her into a deeper issue.

c: Right.

lrc: That part was really important.

c: Right. I know how to get down to the issue. We hit the issue of trust. That was a biggie. I just didn't know where to go from there.

lrc: I think if you would take that last piece, Cate, absolutely this tape would be an A tape, and it would be effective and intentional and efficient.

c: Uh-huh.

lrc: So, just a few minutes left. Give me one thing that you will take from supervision today.

c: Well—

lrc: That you can use with Susan when you see her next.

c: It is, as we've been discussing: it is further understanding of how to move into the process.

lrc: Uh-huh.

c: And I think I would be able to do more process therapy with her.

lrc: Take her to that next level.

c: Exactly.

lrc: And, Cate, the big piece for me is that oftentimes the confrontation piece might have something to do with you. Which is don't be afraid to tell her what you think. You've got the rapport, and if you are willing to do that, you become more effective. That's the piece that I got out of supervision today. So I appreciate the fact that you are letting me do supervision with you today.

c: Thank you.

lrc: You are certainly welcome, Cate, and I will see you in class tomorrow.

c: Tomorrow.

lrc: Thanks, Cate. I know how busy you are. Thanks so very much.

c: It's been my pleasure.

lrc: See you later. Thanks.

Summary

Observing interview tapes and analyzing case presentations are essential to the growth of novice helping professionals. There are other integrative and/or competency-based supervision models that can be used to do just that; however, the microcounseling supervision model (MSM) can be a supervisory method for assisting supervisors and supervisee in naturally strengthening skills. MSM can be used to assist in building a foundation necessary for effective counseling and developmental growth. It provides building blocks for better understanding of basic attending behaviors and influencing skills through the three stages of the MSM: identification, classification, and processing of counseling skills.

The Counseling Interview Rating Form assists in developing a system for reciprocal supervision where supervisees, colleagues, and instructors can offer constructive feedback. This begins a "magic dance" of supervision, where an easy and dynamic flow can encourage supervisees to be receptive to new ideas and interventions. The CIRF not only reviews and teaches how to classify specific skills and behaviors but how to evaluate their intention as well. Finally, the counseling interview rating form assists in examining whether the goals of each interview stage are being achieved. If supervisors and supervisees practice using the MSM and the CIRF, the natural flow of microcounseling supervision will be experienced.

Chapter Seven Final Discussion Questions

1. Based on Cate's supervision questions and her case presentation, how was the microcounseling supervision model the best model selection? Why was it chosen as the best-fit model? _____

   _____

   _____

   _____

2. Of the three MSM components (Reviewing Skills with Intention, Classifying Skills with Mastery, and Summarizing and Processing Supervisory Needs), which component currently helps you understand your supervision concerns?

   _____

   _____

   _____

3. Imagine yourself as a supervisee and supervisor using the microcounseling supervision model. What would be the advantages and disadvantages for you in either role?

   _____

   _____

   _____

   _____

References

Baker, S. B., & Daniels, T. (1989). Integrating research on the microcounseling program: A meta-analysis. *Journal of Counseling Psychology, 36*, 213–222.

Daniels, T. (2002). Microcounseling research: What over 450 data-based studies reveal. In A. Ivey, M. Ivey, & R. Marx (Eds.), *Leader guide to intentional interviewing and counseling.* Pacific Grove, CA: Brooks/Cole.

Haynes, R., Corey, G., & Moulton, P. (2003). *Clinical supervision in the helping professions: A practical guide.* Pacific Grove, CA: Brooks/Cole.

Ivey, A. E., & Ivey, M. B. (2003). *Intentional interviewing and counseling: Facilitating client development in a multicultural society* (5th ed.). Pacific Grove, CA: Brooks/Cole.

Ivey, A. E., Normington, C. J., Miller, C., Morrill, W., & Haase, R. (1968). Microcounseling and attending behavior: An approach to prepracticum counselor training. *Journal of Counseling Psychology, 15*, 1–12.

Lambert, M. J., & Ogles, B. M. (1997). The effectiveness of psychotherapy supervision. In C. E. Watkins, Jr. (Ed.), *The handbook of psychotherapy supervision* (pp. 421–446). New York: Wiley.

Miller, C., Morrill, W., & Uhlemann, M. (1970). An experimental study of pre-practicum training in communicating test results. *Counselor Education and Supervision, 9*, 171–177.

Norcross, J. C., & Halgin, R. P. (1997). Integrative approaches to psychotherapy supervision. In C. E. Watkins Jr. (Ed.), *Handbook of psychotherapy integration* (pp. 203–222). New York: Basic Books.

Russell-Chapin, L. A. (2007). Supervision: An essential for professional counselor development. In J. Gregoire & C. M. Jungers (Eds.), *The counselor's companion: What every beginning counselor needs to know* (pp. 79–80.) Mahwah, NJ: Lawrence Erlbaum.

Russell-Chapin, L., & Ivey, A. (2004a). Microcounselling supervision model: An innovative approach to supervision. *Canadian Journal for Counselling, 7*, 165–176.

Russell-Chapin, L., & Ivey, A. (2004b). *Your supervised practicum and internship: Field resources for turning theory into practice.* Pacific Grove: CA,Brooks/Cole.

Russell-Chapin, L. A., & Sherman, N. E. (2000). The counseling interview rating form: A teaching and evaluation tool for counselor education. *British Journal of Guidance and Counselling, 28*, 115–124.

Scissons, E. H. (1993). *Counseling for results: Principles and practices of helping.* Pacific Grove, CA: Brooks/Cole.

Stoltenberg, C. D. (2008). Supervision. In F. T. L. Leong (Ed.), *Encyclopedia of counseling: Volume one: Changes and challenges for counseling in the 21st century.* Thousand Oaks, CA: Sage.

Interpersonal Process Recall

Interpersonal Process Recall

Borders and Leddick (1998) conducted a national survey of counselor educators and found interpersonal process recall (IPR) to be one of two distinct methods used during supervision courses. The reason this may be true is that IPR creates a supervision environment where supervisees can safely analyze their communication styles and strategies. Kagan believed that most people act diplomatically and often do not say what they mean or feel. In supervision, the supervisor encourages the supervisee to reflect and interpret the experience in the counseling session (Kagan, 1976, 1980).

Historically the interpersonal process recall training model began using the psychoanalytic modeling approach of having counselors in training observe a master counselor conduct counseling interviews. After the session, the expert counselor would express his feelings, thoughts, and intentional behaviors. The student would then mimic the same skills and process his or her feelings, thoughts, and intentional behaviors (Baker, Daniels, & Greeley, 1990; Crews, Smith, Smaby, Maddux, Torres-Rivera, Casey, & Urbani, 2005). This was the beginning of the IPR approach to supervision.

The best way to conduct IPR supervision is to view a videotape of a counseling session and simply stop the tape at any time to discuss essential personal and/or counseling issues. In this manner, supervisees have the opportunity to increase self-awareness and process the relationship dynamics with the client and the supervisor (Haynes, Corey, & Moulton, 2003). The rules of IPR suggest that both the supervisee and supervisor may stop the tape at any given time. The one who stops the interview is the one who speaks first. If the supervisee speaks first, then it is up to the supervisor to give the supervisee enough time and space to reflect options and possibilities (Bernard & Goodyear, 1992).

Discussion Question 1

What do you foresee as the possible IPR benefits to a supervisee? _____

_____

_____

_____

_____

_____

OVERVIEW

Many supervision sessions require videotaping of counseling interviews or conducting counseling sessions in an actual live observation setting. Interpersonal process recall (IPR), developed by Norm Kagan, is an approach that is widely used by many supervisors (Haynes, Corey, & Moulton, 2003). This supervision approach allows supervisees to safely analyze their thoughts and feelings about the counseling interview.

GOALS

- Discover methods for using IPR with videotapes, live supervision, or after the counseling session
- Understand the types of questions that can be utilized with IPR

Often supervisees will express appreciation during supervision for the immediate and timely feedback. There seems to be a better comprehension of the skills and feedback when visually stopping the videotape and discussing intentional feeling, thoughts, and behaviors. It was the work of Norm Kagan and Allen Ivey that inspired the development of the micro-counseling supervision model. Using the Counseling Interview Rating Form (CIRF) while videotaping is just another extension of Kagan's work.

Discussion Questions 2

1. What type of feedback do you want as a supervisee? _____

_____

_____

_____

_____

_____

2. What type of feedback do you want as a supervisor? _____

_____

_____

_____

_____

_____

3. How do you best receive feedback? Directly? Gently? It is best received when you ask for it? Describe. _____

_____

_____

_____

_____

_____

IPR Leads and Questions

Kagan called the good supervisor an "inquirer." Study the following list to see the questions and leads that could be asked while using the interpersonal process recall method (Bernard & Goodyear, 1992. p. 102).

Leads That Inspire Affective Exploration

- Did you want to express that feeling at any time?
- What were your thoughts, feelings, and reactions?

- What did you do about that feeling you had?
- What do those feelings mean to you?

Leads That Check Out Unstated Agendas

- If you had more time, where would you have liked to have gone?
- What would you like to have said to her or him at this point?
- What had that meant to you?
- What's happening here?

Leads That Encourage Cognitive Examination

- Did the equipment affect you in any way?
- What would you like to have said at this point?
- What thoughts were you having about the other person at that time?
- How do you think the client was seeing you at this point?

Leads That Get at Images

- Were there any pictures, images, or memories flashing through your mind then?
- How do you imagine the client was reacting to you?
- Had you any ideas about what you wanted to do with that?
- Where had that put you in the past?

Leads That Explore Mutual Perceptions between Client and Counselor

- What messages do you think she or he was trying to give you?
- How do you think he or she felt about talking with you at this point?
- Do you think your description of the moment would correspond with your client's description?
- Was the client giving you any clues as to how she or he was feeling?

Leads That Help Search Out Expectations

- Were you expecting anything from your client at that point?
- Did you sense that the client had any expectations of you at that point?
- What was it like for you in your role as counselor?
- What message did you want to give the client? What prevented you from doing so?

Discussion Question 3

Which of the above inquiry categories would be easiest and most effective for you to ask? Might your selection have something to do with your own personality?_____

_____

_____

_____

_____

Basic Tenet

- Supervisees need an environment where they can safely analyze their communication styles and strategies.

When to Use

- If a supervisee seems to be stuck in the counseling interview, this method allows for safe, immediate feedback and a chance to reflect on the counseling experience.

Supervisor's Roles and Behaviors

- Stop the videotape at any time to discuss essential personal and/or counseling issues. If a videotape is not available, lead the supervision session with needed questions.

Supervisor's Emphasis and Goals

- The main goal is to stop a counseling videotape or supervisory session and use the skill of immediacy to gently discover counseling blocks, styles, and experiences.

Supervisee's Growth Area

- The supervisee has immediate feedback to assist in safely understanding the strengths and liabilities of the counseling interview.

Limitations

- This supervision approach is best used with video or digital recordings, so the supervisor can start and stop the interview when processing is required. However, a variation of IPR can be used without recordings, by asking the supervisee to recall how he or she felt at that moment.
- This model may not be comprehensive enough alone to meet all the supervisee's needs.

DVD Supervisory Question

This supervisory question suggests that the supervisee needs to take the time to reflect on personal clinical skills and attitudes. The question is "How can I become more effective and clear in my lead, open-ended questions? Lack of clarity often makes me feel less confident and secure in my counseling direction."

Supervision with the Case of Chaka

As Lori listened to Chaka's supervision question and watched the videotape, it was clear that Chaka had the needed counseling skills. However, she was seeking supervision to help her with her confidence levels. Using interpersonal process recall (IPR) seemed like a natural supervision approach to use with Chaka. The first modeling strategy was to build rapport with Chaka until she was comfortable enough to self-disclose. Chaka easily talked about her job and history at the high school. Lori then moved into IPR by asking Chaka targeted questions.

DVD Transcripts from the Case of Chaka

LRC = Lori Russell-Chapin
   C = Chaka

LRC: Thank you so very much for meeting with me today and joining me in supervision. I know that you are a very busy school counselor, and so let's go ahead and get started. I also know that you are having a day off today. That was timely on my part, wasn't it?

C: Yes. Definitely.

LRC: Why don't we start, Chaka, by having you introduce yourself and tell me a little bit about you and where you are in your career, and we'll go from there.

C: My name is Chaka Gibson and I'm a guidance counselor at Woodruff High School. I recently graduated from the program at Bradley this May. Last May.

LRC: It's almost—we're going on a year.

C: Almost a year.

LRC: A whole year.

C: Very excited about that.

LRC: So, Chaka, when you left the program, you took your National Certified Counseling Exam.

C: Yes.

LRC: So you're a National Certified Counselor.

C: Yes, I am.

LRC: And then did you send your scores into the state to get licensed as a counselor?

C: I've done that. I haven't gotten any results back yet.

LRC: So you've taken the test. Oh, you've already taken the test?

C: Yes. I've taken the test.

LRC: But you haven't gotten the results, correct?

C: Well, I got the results. I did pass but—

LRC: Congratulations.

C: Thanks. Thank you.

LRC: There never was a doubt in my mind.

C: Yes. I passed everything and I'm just waiting for my certification.

LRC: To get the actual license that you hang up in your office.

C: Exactly.

LRC: I think, Chaka, that's so important because, you know, a lot of people say as a school counselor that maybe you don't need to be licensed. Because you are not out there seeing a population as a private practice, but to me it just tells the consumer, "I've jumped through all these hoops and I'm a licensed professional counselor."

C: Exactly.

LRC: Now, will you ever consider becoming a licensed clinical professional counselor?

C: I've considered it. I'm not sure where I am with that right now. Right now I'm really happy as a school counselor where I am.

LRC: You never know.

C: You never know.

LRC: That's very cool. Well, tell me a little bit before we get into your case with Michael. Tell me a little bit about what you are doing. What kind of responsibilities you're doing as a school counselor?

C: Well, my responsibilities as a school counselor are—basically I'm a guidance counselor. I guide the students to what they want to do at a post-secondary level. Right now I work with scholarships. I'm the scholarship coordinator. I am on the advisory team at the Urban League. I work with the Upward Bound Program at ICC in the College Yes Program. I'm going to be doing—I do a lot of the testing as well. So, there's a variety of duties that I have. Right now I am letter recommendation writing.

LRC: I bet because everyone is getting ready for college.

C: Oh, my goodness, yes. So that's been one of the main things that I have been doing and just getting kids to apply for scholarships has been really difficult for me.

LRC: You sound like you are very busy.

C: Oh, definitely yes.

LRC: And yet you also have a sparkle in your eye like, "This is a job I really enjoy."

C: It is. I really enjoy what I do. Having graduated from Woodruff, I've been in the kids—

LRC: Oh, you did?

C: Yes. Yes.

LRC: You know the system and you probably know the teachers?

C: Yes. Oh yes. And it's really hard for me to go back and to call them by their first names. I still haven't gotten used to that, so they like it.

LRC: Do they call you Miss Gibson?

C: Yes, they do. Yes, they do. And so it's really kind of difficult for me, but just having been there, it seems like I have a connection with the school and with the students, so I am able to relate more with them in that aspect.

LRC: They are so lucky to have you. Well, I suppose it wasn't luck. They chose you on purpose, but I think it's wonderful that you're there. My last question—we'll get into supervision again—and what is the total population at Woodruff?

C: We have now approximately 900 or so students.

LRC: And how many guidance counselors?

C: We have three guidance counselors and a special ed coordinator.

LRC: Wonderful. So—I mean, to me there needs to be more—but at least it sounds like the students have a chance to get the resources that they might need.

C: Definitely.

LRC: Well, thank you again, Chaka, for joining me.

C: Thank you.

LRC: Tell me a little bit about the case that you are bringing to me in supervision today.

C: The case that I'm bringing to you, I did this during my internship; I was working with a couple of students. One in particular is Michael, which you—

LRC: Saw on the tape.

C: Yes. He is a junior during the taping. A 17-year-old who's just having problems with time management and a whole lot of issues on his faith, and he's not really sure how to delineate responsibilities on all the things that he has going on.

LRC: And you told me earlier though, that when I was watching your tape that—that at Woodruff they assign all the different counselors. Is it alphabetical?

C: Yes.

LRC: It is alphabetical.

C: Yes. Yes. It's divided up A–G and that's the head counselor, Mrs. Wigginstaff. Then myself, I'm H–O. And Mr. McKenna, who also graduated from the program—he's P–Z.

LRC: Okay. That's wonderful. So Michael came to you because he's, like, your charge?

C: Uh-huh.

LRC: Like if you have any questions or comments, this is the person you should be going to?

C: Yes.

LRC: And so, first of all, I have to stop you and ask you: you have consent to talk about Michael?

C: Yes, I do have consent.

LRC: In written and verbal consent from Michael. Again, I'd ask you if you can—and I think let's go over the diagnosis, if you can. On Axis I, Chaka—and you can look at your notes if you have them—Axis I diagnosis. What would be the presenting problem that Michael brings to you in counseling?

C: It's stress. All of the things that he has going on has provided a high level of stress for him, so basically I want to work with him on dealing with the stress that he has.

LRC: And then—I watched the tapes—there are some things, like he's balancing a job?

C: Uh-huh.

LRC: He's trying to do well in school?

C: Correct.

LRC: He's trying to have some fun I if remember him saying?

C: Exactly.

LRC: He's now trying to get things together for an internship?

C: Yes.

LRC: And move onto college, so he has a lot's of things going on in his life.

C: Correct.

LRC: That's Axis I diagnosis. Axis II Personality Disorder?

C: No, there were none.

LRC: It almost sounds like with Axis I, we're dealing with V codes as well. There's not a lot of problems in Michael's life.

C: Right.

LRC: Severe problems but more V codes and peaks on the adjusting level. So Axis II. How about Axis III, which is medical concerns?

C: There were no medical concerns that I saw.

LRC: That you saw. Certainly how it relates to that. Axis IV Psychosocial Stressors?

C: It was basically the time management. Not being able to delineate a time. The things that he has going on at home, like just strained relationships with a stepfather and a younger brother who also attends Woodruff.

LRC: Sibling relationships.

C: Sibling relationships. Definitely.

LRC: As well as parental.

C: Definitely. He was having a few problems in a couple of his classes. One of the classes in particular that he was having problems in. So all those things just combined together had a high-level effect on the stress level that he had.

LRC: And how about Axis V, which would be the GAF score?

C: The GAF score. I rated him probably at about an 85 or so because he's really functioning pretty well. It's just a few minor adjustments that we could make, and that was my goal during the session is to get the GAF score up a little higher.

LRC: Because when I watched the tape, it looked like he was relating to you, Chaka. He looked like he just had so much going for him.

C: Uh-huh.

LRC: And it was nice for him to have someone he could just come and talk to.

C: Right.

LRC: Let me go back a little bit to something, and then we'll get into your supervisory questions. I thought it was really interesting, Chaka, at Woodruff High School—what do you think the ethnic degree is? How many kids are African American? Hispanic? Caucasians? What do you think there?

C: Well, If I remember correctly, we have a really, really high minority population there. I would say—and this is just a guesstimate—about 85 percent are minorities.

LRC: Okay.

C: And of that 85 percent, maybe way over half are African American.

LRC: Because what I noticed, Chaka—and help me out if this is not accurate—but I noticed that because Michael is also African American, that there was a connection to you.

C: Uh-huh.

LRC: And I would guess that he really appreciates the fact that you came from Woodruff. I mean, you know what this is about, and when you talk about a teacher and just say, "You know, you need to get this homework in." You know what you're talking about. I think I could instantly see that kind of connection. What about—what do you do, though, when the student that you are seeing is not African American? Let's say they're Hispanic or Caucasian. What do you do with the differences between the two of you?

C: Well, what I was able to do, which really, really helped me with the Hispanic population is, I was able to do some student teaching there as well.

LRC: I didn't know that.

C: Yes. Yes and I substituted in the ESL, English as a Second Language, class, and I got to know some of those students pretty well and so they knew when I got to their class—I let them know who I was and that I came from Woodruff and that I can understand how it feels to be frustrated about some things and being a minority. So I explained those things to them, and they really related to me, so now when they some to me for sessions, they can talk to me and they feel comfortable with me. So, I was able to build rapport with them. The Hispanic population as well as with the Caucasian population, because I served in some regular of their classes as well.

LRC: But it looks to me like you've done your homework. Like you know that you have to up front address these differences.

C: Definitely.

LRC: And say, "Here it is." And they got to know you in a student–teacher kind of manner, and now they see you in the hall and it's sounds like it's a really nice match.

C: It really is. It really is.

LRC: Chaka, let's go to your supervisory question then. With this tape with Michael, what do you think you need most out of supervision today?

C: What I need most is help with my lead questions. Sometimes I want to be able to be more clear, and more clear and effective in the lead questions. Lead opened-ended questions that I ask. Sometimes I get confused and I feel there are sometimes that I am unclear.

LRC: Okay. And a couple of things that I noticed when I watched the tape, before I even knew the supervisory question, there were a few times that you did dual questions. Like you'd ask a great question. but it was like you didn't know it was a great question, so you'd ask him another question, and the look on the student's face was, "What? What are you talking about?"

C: Exactly. Yes.

LRC: So that's what you're trying to get out of supervision.

C: Correct.

LRC: Well, I've been trying to look at the supervisory question and then base—then based upon that, Chaka, pick a model of supervision I think would be helpful. And what I'd dually do with you—and most people do this when they have the luxury of having a videotape—is, I'd have the videotape right here and we'd watch it from beginning to end.

C: Right.

LRC: And at some point, the viewers of our interview will actually get to watch your videotape, but for today what I would like to do is, I think I would like to focus on—and I'll share this with you: it's really not a supervision model. I've done four different supervision models this afternoon, but this one is more of a videotape processing method.

C: Okay.

LRC: I think what I'll do is I'll go through the tenets with you.

C: Okay.

LRC: And then we're going to ask some specific questions. But the basic tenet of this videotaping process method is that the supervisee needs an environment where they can safely analyze their communication styles and strategies.

C: Okay.

LRC: The example of this kind of method comes from Norm Kagan, and he developed it in the 1980s, a long time ago, something called interpersonal process recall, or IPR. I know you all did that in practicum and internship. So, the idea behinds Kagan's IPR is he says, "You know, sometimes in supervision, it's like we do in counseling: you just say what you think they want to hear just to get it over with, so I can leave their office and get out of there." Kagan's saying, "You know, what I really need to do is provide a really safe place where we can analyze that here." And to do that, the best way to do that is to stop the tape and immediately say, "What's happening right now?" It's that immediacy piece in counseling. So, today when I saw your tape, there was one point that we were looking for that was so wonderful, Chaka, because you have, I'd have to say, very insightful open-ended questions, and Michael answered them. He knew exactly. But it almost felt like there was a point where, in your head—and I don't know if this is true—but in your head you went, "Okay, I don't what to do next."

C: Yeah.

LRC: And so you asked this question, and he really did gaze at you kind of like, "I'm not sure what I'm supposed to say. So that specifically, that moment on the tape, is when you feel sometimes that you get lost.

C: Definitely.

LRC: Is that accurate?

C: Yes.

LRC: Well, then let's do that. We're going to talk a little bit about IPR.

C: Okay.

LRC: When I would choose this method would be when the supervisee seems to be stuck in the counseling interview and then, by stopping the tape, I can give you some immediate feedback. But a lot of times people in supervision don't have a videotape. I mean, I'm a fan of videotaping, but everybody gets kind of nervous about it. But you don't even need to have it. If we don't have it, I can still stop and say, "What are you doing right now?" So, one of the things that I would do is, since we don't have a videotape, I'm just going to lead you, Chaka, with some questions I think might try to answer your supervisor question.

C: Okay.

LRC: There are some other people who have done some work with Kagan's material; it's Bernard and Goodyear. They have about twenty, I think, great questions. So I'm going to ask you a couple questions.

C: Okay.

LRC: At the very moment on the videotape that we stopped this morning, where you asked some dual questions—I'll even take that from you—you asked dual questions and you get that puzzled look from Michael. What specifically, Chaka, were you thinking and feeling right at that moment?

C: I was nervous and first of all, I was confused because I didn't know what I was trying. I knew what I wanted to say, but it wouldn't come out, so I was a little bit confused, and then I became nervous and then I lost confidence in the things that I was going to say. Even though I thought they were good things I was going to say, when I couldn't get it out, I lost confidence and became nervous.

LRC: Chaka, when you lost confidence, whether it's in a counseling situation or a teaching situation or just a personal situation, what happens to you behaviorally?

C: Wow. Well, first of all, the expression shows on my face like, "What now?"

LRC: Oh no.

C: So it shows on my face, and then I have to start thinking about it and trying to just process everything, and when I do that, I feel like I'm losing my audience or I'm losing the client, so it's kind of difficult to draw them back in after I lose that.

LRC: So it's almost like—this may not be quite the right word—but kind of a frantic feeling.

C: That's it.

LRC: And then, when I'm thinking about my frantic feelings and thoughts, I've lost my audience. Well, let me back up for a second. Do you think that Michael has ever felt like that? Do you think your client has ever felt like that?

C: I think sometimes just by looking at his face I would say so, but he made me feel comfortable, and even though he was confused, I could see that he was still there with me. I didn't totally lose him, so I think by establishing the rapport with him early on in our sessions and developing a good counselor relationship with him, I was able to keep him there. Even though it was difficult for me and I was even more nervous than he was.

LRC: See, I think you hit on something that was really valuable for you, Chaka, which is, I think Michael—I think all of us have felt like you have felt. Even today, doing this, it was like I slipped on a couple words and it was like, "Oh Lord, come on." But it's like everybody does that, Chaka. So I think you've got to know that universality is there. Everybody has that feeling. That's the first thing I think you have to know. Secondly, I think it's really important for you to figure out "If that's how I feel and this is what I'm thinking, why not say it?"

c: Okay.

lrc: So what—if you could—and this takes courage—then we'll talk about how this whole thing works—but if you have the courage to stop because you realize that "I'm feeling frantic" and you say this to Michael, what would you say? And you can't do this wrong.

c: I would probably say, "I think I need to regroup. Let me regroup, Michael, so give me just a second to regroup and get my thoughts correct."

lrc: I think that would be perfect, Chaka. I think that would be great. Or even to say—which yours is a much nicer way to say it—I've even said in therapy before, "You know what? I got lost. I lost my train of thought." What do you think that impact would be on Michael or any client if you had the courage to say those things?

c: I think they would respect me more because they know that you are human and you're just like them.

lrc: Exactly.

c: And everybody make mistakes and everybody needs a chance to regroup and to start over.

lrc: So they think we're human, then we're also modeling what, Chaka? What are we modeling? And you can't be wrong on this one either.

c: Oh boy.

lrc: I'm going to stop you right now. Did it just happen to you? Did you just feel like, "I don't know what to say?"

c: Right.

lrc: Then that's what I want you to say to me. Say, "You know what, Laurie? I don't know. I don't have an answer." Try that.

c: I don't know. I don't have an answer for that.

lrc: Okay. That's okay, because I put you on the spot, so that makes some sense. Now, tell me what happens when you have the courage to say—on a tape no less—"I don't have an answer."

c: It made me feel a little better because now you know where I am at that point, so you're not trying to wonder what's going on in my mind.

lrc: What's wrong with her? Exactly. I know what's going on and honestly—here's the really tough question—and by being honest and genuine, was your anxiety level reduced?

c: Yes.

lrc: Yes. I think so. And if we can model that to a client or to anybody, a student as well as a teacher, I think it makes them say, "Hey, that person is human. I do respect them more and, you know, I could try that. Next time, I'll try that."

c: Right.

lrc: I want you to start—when we get into counseling and we're trying to answer your supervisory question, Chaka—don't be afraid to make a mistake, because I want to go here a little bit with you. This is the interpersonal process recall. I'm trying to get you to think about why you do the things you do and how you do them.

c: Okay.

LRC: If you could admit to people as a school guidance counselor, "I don't have all the answers," what does that do to you and everyone around you?

C: I think by saying that, it lets them know that this is a learning process and we're all learning together, so—

LRC: I love what you just said: "This isn't just my imparting knowledge to you. This is, we're learning together as a unit."

C: Yes.

LRC: So, whenever we get lost or I get nervous or I get frustrated, we can stop the process and we can say whatever we want to say. But in any way, Chaka, when you do that, do you feel as if somehow you're not quite as powerful? Or you're not quite as expert a counselor if you do that?

C: I don't feel that I'm as powerful. My biggest thing when I do that is because the age difference between me and the students that I counsel is not so big.

LRC: What is it exactly? How old are you?

C: Probably about—I'm 30.

LRC: Okay. They're 18. They think you're 22 or something.

C: Exactly. Which I don't tell them otherwise. But when I do that, it seems like they maybe won't take me as seriously because I'm so young. So, I want to have all the answers but I know that I don't, so what I try to do in instances like that is just get on the Internet or pick up the phone and give them the answers that they need, or I simply tell them that I'll get back with them.

LRC: But, Chaka, I think you said something else that was really important, which is that "I'm afraid that they're not going to think that I have as much expertise as possible." One of the things that I think you need to know is that it's okay to say to people, "I don't know."

C: Right.

LRC: Or, "I don't have the answer." What I even do when I teach at Bradley with a student—when you ask me a question and I don't know, I won't fake it. Because I believe most people know when we're faking it.

C: Right.

LRC: Don't you think?

C: Yes. I do.

LRC: So I won't fake and I'll say, "That is an incredible question. Here's what I want you to do. I want you to go home and research it, and I'm going to go home tonight and research it, and when I see you again, let's get together collectively and see what we can come up with." Because then, again, you are teaching them how to get to the resource.

C: Exactly.

LRC: Not that we all have the answers. So, Chaka, you just hit another part for you. That's one of reasons this is your supervisor question. "Why I struggle sometimes. Because I'm afraid they won't think—they won't take me seriously."

C: Exactly.

LRC: But I think if you can teach them—it's a wonderful old—and I never give it justice—it's a wonderful old phrase about, "If I give someone a fish, they're going to eat for a day, but if I teach them how to fish, they can eat for a lifetime."

C: Yes.

LRC: That's what you're doing. I think you're teaching them how to deal with anxiety.

C: That's right. That's a good point.

LRC: How to deal with the fact that "I don't know sometimes. I don't have the answers."

C: Right.

LRC: And then what it does is, it says, "You can find the answers. I can find the answers." So I think that's one of the ways we can help you with your supervisor question. Let's take a look at another one. We'll just do one more.

C: Okay.

LRC: We just hit this one. You know, what were you thinking and feeling at the time. We talked about why—what stops you from doing that. Let's take a look at another great question—I thought—I thought this was a fun one; here's another great question: Were there any pictures, images, or memories flashing through your mind when Michael gives you that, "What are you talking about, Chaka?" Any pictures? Memories? Anything flashing through your mind?

C: Yes. One of the things that—when I'm in that position, it takes me back to being in the classroom. Whether it's at Bradley or in high school. It just takes me back to being in front of a class when I have—when I'm talking in front of the class—and what I want to say doesn't come out.

LRC: Yeah.

C: So everybody's looking at me like . . .

LRC: It's the same thing we just talked about.

C: Yes. And so I get nervous and I, like, shut down kind of.

LRC: Well, Chaka, here's what I want to do with the few remaining minutes we have in supervision today. I want to suggest that if you're willing to look at these images, that could help you—the image of Chaka when you get frustrated or anxious. Describe them to me.

C: Scared. Kind of like a little girl who is lost.

LRC: Yes.

C: And that's exactly what I feel like.

LRC: A little girl who is lost.

C: Uh-huh.

LRC: I want to go back—and I'm teaching kind of an imaging technique that I think you can use, and I'm going to try to anchor it so when you leave here today, you'll have a resource. A new resource that you can have, but you can give it to anybody else. We talked about this image in your head is, "I'm a lost child. Lost little girl wandering around going, 'Help me. Someone help me.'" Talk to me about in a moment in your life, though, when you were a 30-year-old female who is powerful and confident. Tell me about that person.

C: Just on top. Just has knowledge of what she is talking about and just very confident, and everyone is going to look to me as a person with the knowledge, who can help, and I felt that way quite a bit.

LRC: What was really interesting, Chaka, though, is when you were talking about that person . . .

C: My body . . .

LRC: You sat up like this. You know. And your voice was stronger. Everything about that was different than the lost little girl. Well, here's what I want you to imagine if you can. Can you imagine for me that lost little girl? What would your 30-year-old do—and how old is your little girl, by the way, who is lost?

C: Probably an 8-year-old.

LRC: Okay. So we're talking like second or third grade, and she is really lost and scared. What would the 30-year-old Chaka do? What would she say to the 8-year-old Chaka who is lost?

C: That it will be okay. That I would help her find who she's looking for or just guide her out of that terrifying situation.

LRC: In your mind's eye, can you imagine maybe taking her hand and giving her a big hug?

C: Yes. Definitely.

LRC: That's what I want to leave you with today, Chaka. I want to see if you can imagine the 9-year-old holding hands with the 30-year-old and saying, "We can do this together because"—here's the piece I think is interesting about this; you know this as a counselor. What are the benefits of anxiety?

C: That you learn from them and you grow stronger. They make you stronger.

LRC: And they keep us safe. Right?

C: They keep us safe.

LRC: So I don't want him to get rid of it totally. I just want to build on its resources. So you're not saying to the 9-year-old, "Go away." Or to the 8-year-old girl, "Go away." Let's join forces—and I think that's facilitated anxiety—let's join forces so we can work together as this confident sitting-up-straight person who may not have all the answers, but "I think I know how to get where I need to go." Does that part make sense?

C: That makes a lot of sense.

LRC: Tell me what you looked like. My last little piece. When you were 9, what kind of hair did you have? Is it long?

C: Two little pony tails.

LRC: Pigtails? Oh I love it.

C: Yes. And I always had barrettes and little bows on them, so yeah.

LRC: So you've moved from that to this sophisticated woman who doesn't have all the answers but is quite confident.

C: Yes.

LRC: It's pretty nice, isn't it?

C: It's very nice.

LRC: So, let me ask you this: What did you do? What do we take today? This is the interpersonal process we call method, Chaka. What can you take from this method that can help you next time you see Michael or the next time you're standing in front of a group of students?

C: Well, that it's okay to not have all the answers. It's okay to say that I don't have all the answers, but let's work together to try to find what we're looking for. It's okay to give responsibility to the client as well, and that makes what you're trying to do even stronger.

LRC: Doesn't it? It's even a better outcome. Isn't it?

C: Definitely. It puts them in charge of it as well. "I'm not just giving you what I think it should be. You have some kind of responsibility in it as well."

LRC: And, Chaka—because I'll end this today with this: you have an incredible responsibility as a school counselor.

C: Definitely.

LRC: But the burden shouldn't be all on you.

C: Exactly.

LRC: And that what I love about this shared kind of community is that I can share this and I can teach people how to find resources.

C: Right.

LRC: Then your 9-year-old little girl is okay. She's giving you wonderful hints, but she doesn't have to do this by herself.

C: Exactly.

LRC: So, did you get out of supervision today what you needed?

C: Yes, I did. Today, I think, from what you told me, I really can see myself using everything you told me when I go back to work and in life in general, so I really appreciate that.

LRC: Chaka, thank you because I know how busy you are, and I just hope you'll—of course, my little piece is, I hope you will think about getting that LCPC and continuing supervision. I think it helps us all. And the piece I don't think I told you was that I started going. I'm now in supervision and I've been doing therapy for 29 years. I love it, so I hope you'll continue to do it. Thank you so much, Chaka, for talking to me. It's so good to see you again too.

C: Thank you.

LRC: Thanks so much. See you later.

Summary

Using targeted questions in supervision allows the supervisor to assist the supervisee in better understanding the hows and whys that occurred in the counseling session. Often supervisees leave the supervision session with additional clarity of personal issues that may impede counseling success and outcomes.

Chapter Eight Final Discussion Questions

1. Was IPR a good model to fit the supervision question? How was this supervision session successful in answering the question? _____

_____

_____

_____

_____

2. If you could use the IPR supervision method of viewing videotaped sessions, what would the benefits be of this supervision model? _____

_____

_____

_____

_____

3. Select three IPR questions from the list in this chapter, and imagine how the discussion might develop. _____

_____

_____

_____

_____

_____

References

Baker, S. B., Daniels, T. G., & Greeley, A. T. (1990). Systemic training of graduate-level counselors: Narrative and meta-analytic reviews of three major programs. *The Counseling Psychologist, 18,* 355–421.

Bernard, J. M., & Goodyear, R. K. (1992). *Fundamentals of clinical supervision.* Needham Heights. MA: Allyn and Bacon.

Borders, L. D., & Leddick, G. R. (1998). A nationwide survey of supervisory training. *Counselor Education and Supervision Journal, 27,* 271–283.

Crews, J., Smith, M. R., Smaby, M. H., Maddux, C. D., Torres-Rivera, E., Casey, J., & Urbani, S. (2005). Self-monitoring and counseling skills: Skills-based versus interpersonal process recall training. *Journal of Counseling and Development, 83,* 78–85.

Haynes, R., Corey, G., & Moulton, P, (2003). *Clinical supervision in the helping profession: A practical guide.* Pacific Grove, CA: Brooks/Cole.

Kagan, N. (1976). *Influencing human interaction.* Mason, MI: Mason Media.

Kagan, N. (1980). Influencing human interaction–Eighteen years with IPR. In A. K. Hess (Ed.), *Psychotherapy supervision: Theory, research and practice* (pp. 262–286). New York: Wiley.

Realizing the Many Benefits of Group Supervision

Group Supervision

The primary purpose of group supervision is to provide a rich opportunity for clinical input, continued professional education and skill enhancement, collegial support, and staff development. Imagine the vast array of experience and knowledge in a room filled with a multidisciplinary team of freshly trained and well-seasoned professional counselors, social workers, psychologists, and psychiatrists. Imagine, even further, the value in the participation of many allied professionals, including but not limited to nurses, nutritionists, rehabilitation specialists, and vocational experts. The diversity of professional perspective and theoretical orientation alone can't help but yield a superior advantage in the formulation of an effective treatment plan. In addition, the mere multiplicity of various eyes and ears on a clinical problem would certainly extend any therapist's depth of understanding and potential options for the client's successful treatment. Current research on group supervision will challenge old ideas about supervision and keep the profession growing (Russell-Chapin & Ivey, 2004). Research results have great implications for future direction in supervision. Ray and Altekruse (2000) conducted group supervision research and found that group supervision is not only complementary to individual supervision but actually may be exchanged for individual supervision.

Group supervision is also effective in providing continued professional education and skill development. No single professional can reasonably keep up with the burgeoning literature or specialty certifications that a group of professionals possess. It's not uncommon in group supervision for a participating therapist to share an article reference or explain or even demonstrate a newly learned therapeutic skill. This helps young therapists add to their therapeutic tool kits and mature therapists to refresh their skills as they pass their knowledge on to others.

Perhaps more subtle, but none-the-less more important, is the collegial support and camaraderie that group supervision creates among its participants. It is not easy to be vulnerable with your peers, ask for help, or admit that you are struggling with a case. It's also not easy to risk sharing your ideas, feelings, intuition, and even special expertise with a colleague. What if you embarrass yourself by displaying your inadequacy? What if your input is ignored or, even worse, argued against by another group member? There is much emotional risk in group supervision, but there is even more potential reward when you find direction with a perplexing problem or receive sincere gratitude from a very appreciative colleague. Well-facilitated group supervision has an enormous potential for building collegial support and enhancing overall group morale.

Finally, group supervision offers the opportunity for meaningful staff development. We all started out as rookies with lots of book knowledge and precious little professional experience. Although we may have felt we were well prepared to help our clients, we soon found out that sitting face-to-face with a complex problem we've never seen before or being humbled by a seemingly impossible therapeutic impasse is altogether

OVERVIEW

In the last 15 years, the increased demand for counseling services and the economic impact of limited third-party reimbursement have resulted in extraordinary demands on individual practitioners. Ever-increasing overhead costs, lengthening work schedules, and professional isolation have caused practitioners to consider the many benefits of the group practice model. Along the way, many of them also realized the advantages of consolidating their supervisory needs. Interest in group supervision experienced a remarkable resurgence.

This chapter will outline the purpose of group supervision, its many advantages, and some of its limitations. It will also outline a procedure that can be readily applied to many mental health settings. Special attention will be given to the facilitator's role and the many clinical issues that group supervision sessions can address. Finally, the chapter will close with a brief review of some related but vitally important topics that will explore some of the following questions: Should participation in group supervision be voluntary or mandatory? Should mental health professionals be charged for supervision? What kind of documentation will the facilitator need to keep? How can a group handle an issue involving an impaired therapist? How does group supervision change in various work settings? When is group supervision just not enough?

GOALS

- Identify the advantages and limitations of group supervision
- Offer a basic procedure for group supervision
- Observe a demonstration of group supervision of a supervisor becoming the supervisee

another matter. Group supervision affords us the opportunity to benefit from all the experience of each professional in the group. Chances are, someone has been right where we are, struggled with the same problem, and found a way through it. Someday, we too will be in that experienced position, and then we'll pass our knowledge and experience on to another therapeutic rookie. Thus group supervision is an invaluable source for staff development.

Discussion Question 1

Offer your thoughts about the importance of group supervision to the counseling profession._____

_____

_____

_____

_____

Advantages

The most obvious advantage of group supervision is that it maximizes the resources of experience, time, and support. As noted above, the value of bringing years of professional training and experience into one room and focusing it on one therapist's case simply cannot be duplicated in any other way. The powerful dynamics of group supervision maximize the resources of a group practice.

Group supervision also helps each participant through the miracle of vicarious learning. Even a staff member who remains quiet during group supervision benefits from the information he hears and the support he witnesses between other staff members. The problem the group is discussing today may be the very problem that the therapist will encounter tomorrow. Vicarious learning occurs whether a group supervision participant is presenting a case, helping with a case, or learning through observation of other participants.

Group supervision also allows for multidisciplinary and multitheoretical input. Over time, most therapists tend to favor a certain approach to their therapeutic work. Perhaps they feel most comfortable within a medical model, a developmental approach, a family systems perspective, or a psychodynamic understanding of the client's experience. Perhaps a certain viewpoint better matches their personality. Very often, stepping outside of our own biases, assumptions, and blind spots can help us take a fresh look at our own work with a particular client and allow us to be ultimately more helpful to them.

Group supervision also has the advantage of a few secondary functions of a group practice. It can provide a valuable check-and-balance mechanism on therapists' clinical work. By presenting a case, asking for feedback, and hearing the input from the other participants, both the presenting member and the other group participants can gauge their relative expertise, skill, and ability. This is valuable because it can assist in both the initial case assignment and later in-group referral process. By knowing the relative strengths and limitations of any given member, a better client–therapist match may be made from the start of treatment, and more effective in-group referrals can be facilitated.

Finally, group supervision also has the secondary advantage of setting the values and professional tone of the group practice. Groups who adopt the group supervision model do so with a preference for openness and vulnerability, collaborative learning, and continued personal and professional growth. The value of these is not to be understated; however, they are realized only through the implementation of effective group supervision techniques and a skillful group supervision facilitator.

Discussion Question 2

What will be the major advantages of group supervision to you? _____

_____

_____

_____

_____

Limitations

Group supervision may not be the best choice for all group practices. There are several disadvantages to this approach to supervision. The first is time. Because group practices can vary greatly in their number of members, the time allocated for group supervision must be proportionate to the supervision needs of its members. If too little time is planned, then group members will become frustrated and the depth of meaningful feedback will be limited. Eventually, members may simply choose not to participate or do so only in a limited or less meaningful fashion.

The limitation of time may not hold true for higher education, however. In fact, practicing group supervision in triads allows for more diversity for students and additional time spent in individual supervision for faculty.

Another disadvantage is the need for active participation. Many therapists are by their nature introverted. Others may not feel as confident about sharing their struggles with other group members. Still others may be satisfied sitting on the sidelines and observing. Although this does have the benefit of vicarious education, it may, in time, create an uncomfortable imbalance in group supervision participation. To help guard against this problem, the group may want to rotate case presenters, and the group facilitator may be well advised to solicit everyone's involvement in providing feedback to the presenter. Linton (2003) states that supervisees in group supervision tend to cushion the feedback instead of being open and honest. If this does occur, then the supervisor could make this issue a supervision topic to discuss.

Of a more ominous nature is the possibility that group supervision may uncover underlying dysfunctional group dynamics. Therapists are after all human beings. As such, we bring our own stuff to all the groups in which we are members. Sometimes we too can form unconscious alliances, can triangulate other group members, or even sabotage healthy group interaction through our own projections and unhealthy behavior. If group supervision does uncover underlying dysfunctional group dynamics, perhaps it is in the group's long-term best interests to identify and appropriately deal with them.

A final potential disadvantage of group supervision is the risk for the formation of theoretical camps and resulting turf wars that could monopolize the type and quality of input a presenter might receive or cause the supervision session to descend into a debate on theoretical supremacy. As previously noted, many therapists have their theoretical or specialty-focused preferences. Rather than allow one viewpoint to dominate, it falls upon the group to establish the value of a multidisciplinary and multitheoretical approach and the group facilitator to affirm that value by encouraging a variety of feedback.

Discussion Question 3

Add to our list of limitations. What other limitations might concern you about group supervision? _____

_____

_____

_____

Procedures

For years, the main method of conducting supervision was individual supervision. In 2001, the Council for Accreditation of Counseling and Related Education Programs (CACREP) approved triadic supervision as an additional method of offering supervision. Triadic supervision creates a new system, with usually one supervisor paired with two supervisees (Hein & Lawson, 2008). Within that system, there are numerous methods of conducting supervision. In a study by Nguyen (2004), the differences between a single focus and split focus were examined. Although there were no differences in supervisees' effectiveness between the two types, there was a positive difference in supervisee development with split focus. Single-focus supervision has one supervisee sharing a case(s) for one entire session, whereas split focus has both supervisees offering cases equally during the session.

In another dissertation, Bakes (2005) investigated the supervisory working alliance between the supervisory team, whether individual or triadic. The results suggest that triadic supervision minimizes identification with the supervisor and his or her supervisory perspective but increases the supervisees' understanding of the clients and cases.

Regardless of the type of group supervision, the first task of the group supervision facilitator is to call the session to order. This may take some doing if you have a busy staff. Once it is established who will be attending the day's session, the door to the room is closed and the meeting is not interrupted except for an emergency. Next, the facilitator sets a few ground rules such as confidentiality, the goals of group supervision, and intent to be respectful and helpful to one another. Then the facilitator surveys the group to determine those who would like to present a case and the general theme of each case to be presented. Sometimes a group member will want to present an entire case. Other times only one particular aspect of a case will be presented for discussion. Next, the cases for the supervision agenda are prioritized and discussion begins. It can be useful when prioritizing the cases to be sure to allow enough time for the depth and complexity of the theme to be discussed. This is either determined by experience, or the presenting group member may offer an estimate of how much time he or she will likely need. Brief items are often best addressed first, to clear the slate for the more involved cases. Once completed, it is easier to allocate the remaining time to the group members who have requested more in-depth discussion.

Now the group is ready to focus on each individual case. The presenting member is encouraged to share some background information about the case. This can include demographics, presenting concern, relevant history, family of origin, marital adjustment, risk of abuse, risk of substance abuse, previous treatment, test results, diagnosis, medication, current treatment plan, and response to treatment. Then the facilitator calls for the question "How can we help you?" or "What do you need from us?" or "What do you want out of supervision today?" The facilitator then encourages group discussion. At the initial stage of discussion, the group members readily offer their feedback. A few are often very verbal and others remain quiet. Once the initial discussion seems to slow, additional comments are solicited from the more quiet members. The facilitator may restate some of the comments or summarize the general themes. When the discussion seems to close, the facilitator then checks in with the presenting therapist to verify that she received the feedback she was seeking. If an affirmative answer is received, the discussion proceeds to the next case. If not, the facilitator then requests that the presenter restate or refine her question, and further discussion is facilitated. Discussion continues until the presenter feels sufficient feedback has been provided or until her allotted time has expired.

As the supervision session nears its end, the facilitator asks what each supervisee gained from supervision, summarizes the themes of the day, reviews any follow-up tasks, and sets the next supervision session. All participants are thanked for their participation, and the facilitator makes appropriate notes about the supervision session.

Discussion Question 4

What procedural element, if any, would you add to make the group run more smoothly?

_____

_____

_____

The Facilitator's Role

The primary role of the facilitator is to provide structure for the supervision session. This includes organizing the agenda, managing the time, and maintaining the focus that best seems to meet the presenter's request. The facilitator is also responsible for maintaining an atmosphere that is conducive to open discussion and encourages group member participation. This is not always easy, because some cases will inevitably generate healthy debate, some presenters may express defensiveness, and some feedback may not always be complimentary. It is still vitally important that the facilitator promote an environment that will help group members to speak and case presenters to listen.

New supervision groups, as with other kinds of groups, may initially struggle to achieve a healthy working atmosphere. Although the purpose of a supervision group is usually clear, to aid each other in the provision of effective therapy, members may struggle with establishing appropriate norms and fall into periods of unexpected conflict. It is vital in these situations that the supervision group facilitator take the lead in establishing effective group norms and processing any group conflict that may emerge. If this is not done, the task of effective group supervision will not be accomplished.

Discussion Question 5

Would you imagine that group supervision evolves much like group counseling, where eventually the group members take on much of the facilitator's roles? Discuss. _____

_____

_____

_____

Focus of Group Supervision

The focus of group supervision can take many different forms. The most typical is a case presentation intended to seek input on treatment planning and effective interventions. Just as often, however, a therapist is looking for help with case conceptualization. He understands the presenting concern and the client's symptomology but struggles to understand the underlying dynamics that maintain the client's undesired behavior. The multidisciplinary and multitheoretical strengths of group supervision are often very helpful in enhancing case conceptualization.

Group supervision is also a useful forum for providing case updates. Much can be learned from what went well and what went poorly. Some cases can become exemplars and are great examples to illustrate the utility of a certain technique or intervention strategy. Cases that turn out poorly can also be excellent learning tools. In group supervision, the members can conduct a therapeutic autopsy, reviewing what happened, what did not work, and what might have led to a better outcome.

Group supervision in a community setting has similarities to peer group supervision that recent graduate students have encountered. There are advantages and disadvantages to this type of supervision. A systematic, structured approach seems to alleviate many of the concerns about peer group supervision (Borders, 1991). Granello, Kindsvatter, Granello, Underfer-Babalis, and Hartwig-Moorhead (2008) write that a supervisory peer consultation group also widens and expands critical thinking and case conceptualization skills in each of the team members. A structured peer group format has the following advantages:

- Ensures all members are involved
- Emphasizes focused and objective feedback
- Emphasizes cognitive counseling skills
- Can be used with groups of experienced and inexperienced counselors
- Provides a framework for supervisors
- Teaches an approach for self-monitoring (Fall & Sutton, 2004)

Structured peer group consultation supervision is the type of supervision that is provided in this chapter's DVD demonstration.

Ethical issues are also an important focus of group supervision. Discussions about the risks of dual relationships, involvement of children and family services, duty to warn, confidentiality, client's right to refuse treatment, limits of therapist expertise, and need to refer are only a few of the issues with which group supervision can help.

There are also several counselor issues that group supervision can address. These include countertransference, projection, and other forms of therapeutic bias or distortion that are much more easily seen from outside the therapeutic relationship than within it. Group supervision can provide a safe and helpful environment to identify these dynamics and discuss their resolution.

Sometimes client issues will also affect therapeutic effectiveness. Such considerations as client readiness for change, developmental level of functioning, and sources of client resistance are more readily observable from an outside perspective. In addition, gender, age, and cultural diversity issues can also be explored in supervision. As therapists, we often like to think that we can help everyone who steps through our door, but the truth is we are products of our own gender, age, and cultural background, and perhaps the input from a diverse group of colleagues will help us recognize our limits and/or learn how to more effectively bridge the diversity.

In group supervision, we can also learn new techniques, new skills, and the latest research findings related to our concern. Although our ethics generally compel us to work within the limits of our own expertise, there are many more subtle techniques and skills that we continuously acquire throughout our years of practice. Group supervision can help us learn and apply these techniques while under the supervision of those who possess them. In addition, group supervision can help keep us informed of the latest research pertaining to our area of inquiry. It is very difficult for one individual to keep up with the professional literature, and it's much easier to rely on the collective study of a group of colleagues.

Group supervision can be an invaluable place for learning about the referral sources in your own community. Chances are that many of your more experienced colleagues have great feedback about the many community resources in your area. Whether these are particular individual practitioners, community programs, or even allied professionals, your colleagues know the reputations and can steer you toward the resources that will be most helpful to your clients.

Information about professional development, credentialing, or specialty training is also available from more experienced group supervision members. Who to call, where to pick up an application, necessary requirements, trainers to avoid, and trainers to sign on with—your group supervision members are often a wealthy source of tested professional development information.

Finally, a more mundane but nonetheless very important aspect of any professional's job is information about administrative issues. What forms are used for what purpose? How do I handle the paperwork? What is our policy about this? How do I handle past due accounts with my clients? These are just some of the administrative questions that can be readily answered through group supervision. Why reinvent the wheel when those who designed it are available for your ready consultation?

Discussion Question 6

What are the essential issues that you would like to have addressed in your group supervision? _____

_____

_____

_____

_____

Other Important Issues in Group Supervision

Should participation in group supervision be voluntary or mandatory? Most mental health professional associations recommend that its members be actively involved in supervision. They do not necessarily dictate whether that supervision is individual or group. Most group practices attempt to support this recommendation by encouraging their members to participate in ongoing professional supervision, whether individual or group. There are some professionals who take exception to this, feeling that they have enough experience and training and therefore do not need ongoing supervision. This is a shortsighted view of the role of supervision in clinical practice. The value and benefits of supervision are well established. Supervision is a place to get feedback, receive support, become rejuvenated, and most importantly improve one's therapeutic effectiveness. Group supervision provides the rich, professionally diverse context for this to occur. Although in practice supervision has yet to be mandated, it is one voluntary activity that is essential to guard liability, prevent malpractice, and, more positively, to assure continued development of clinical expertise.

Should participation in group supervision be paid or unpaid? Generally speaking, it is always important to value the professional work of another through reasonable remuneration for services rendered. With the collegial atmosphere of group supervision, the roles of case presenter and feedback provider frequently change within one session. Even the group facilitator, who may not be presenting a case, benefits from the discussion that unfolds. In many ways, all participants of group supervision both contribute to and benefit from it. A common private practice model is that no one is paid for participation in group supervision because no revenue is being generated and all participants receive significant professional benefit. In an agency setting, where staff are paid by salary, group supervision is simply one of the expected job duties, and its remuneration is included in staff salaries. Payment for private group supervision, beyond that offered by an agency or a private practice, is typically paid for by the participants and provided by a facilitator with higher credentials. If all participating parties benefit, perhaps payment is not necessary. Payment is a decision that is best determined by review of the various factors in the practice setting.

Documentation is a very important aspect of both individual and group supervision. As in therapy, where paperwork provides a record of the therapeutic process, supervision documentation provides a record of appropriate professional review. In malpractice liability cases, one of the more common professional mistakes is not to have sought supervisory input into a critical treatment issue. Even when one has sought input, it is typically not sufficient just to report that one spoke with his supervisor. Detailed documentation about the nature of the discussion and the resulting action plan or recommendations is the best evidence to validate appropriate professional practice.

One of the more difficult supervisory issues to address is that of an impaired therapist. The process of group supervision sometimes reveals obvious problems with therapist impairment but more often yields subtle indicators that suggest that a therapist may be practicing with a significant personal impairment. Some examples of common therapist impairments include substance abuse, an untreated mental health problem, or significant personal life stressors such as divorce or close family loss that might emotionally overwhelm a therapist and impede her therapeutic objectivity, judgment, and effectiveness. To avoid an undue defensive reaction from the identified impaired therapist, it may be best to provide constructive feedback first in an individual supervision setting. Once acknowledged and an action plan agreed upon, the matter may be more readily addressed in the group supervision setting. Although it is useful to attend to the collegial impact of therapist impairment in the group setting, it is first necessary for the impaired therapist to be able to accept his impairment and take ownership of his personal recovery plan.

Another important issue in group supervision is how the expectations, focus, and form of supervision may change depending upon the employment setting. Typical settings for mental health services include private practice, school, agency, medical, educational, and business. Each of these settings has a different service population and varies in the type of allied professionals with whom the mental health provider collaborates. The diversity of each of these settings does not allow for a detailed review here, but one illustrative example might help the reader appreciate the necessity of attending to these differences. This example involves differences in the assumptions underlying medical versus traditional mental health settings. Most traditional mental health settings view treatment as primarily a one-to-one relationship between a client and a therapist. Most medical health settings view a client's treatment as a team effort. Both settings operate on different assumptions about confidentiality, the comprehensiveness of treatment, and how authority and accountability are handled within the treatment team. Supervision issues are not only about the client–therapist relationship but likely also include the client's physical and perhaps vocational health needs. The individual therapist is not the primary authority for treatment; a nurse, nutritionist, social worker, physician, psychiatrist, and so forth, together develop and implement the client's treatment plan. And confidentiality is not reserved only for the individual therapist; it is granted to the treatment team. Sensitivity to the demands of different employment settings and modification of group supervision expectations, focus, and form will make group supervision more effective.

The final important issue in group supervision is its insufficiency in providing the depth of case review that is sometimes necessary to effectively assist a presenting therapist or a group of therapists who want feedback. Group supervision time is often limited; the larger the group, the greater the likelihood that some cases will not be sufficiently reviewed. Some groups deal with this by prioritizing the cases to be presented, asking staff to prepare a summary of their case ahead of time, limiting the time each group member has to present, and providing ample individual supervision to follow up on any needs that cannot be addressed in the group session. Still other issues sometimes emerge that call for deeper, more personal reflection, such as those involving transference, countertransference, projection, or parataxic distortion. In a supervision group with strong trust, emotionally secure therapists, and a skillful facilitator, these issues can be successfully addressed. However, sometimes, a therapist may feel inhibited in exploring the personal basis underlying these dynamics in front of her colleagues and would rather, and perhaps more effectively, do so in individual supervision. Group supervision has many advantages, but its limitations must also be noted.

Discussion Question 7

Offer your thoughts and feelings about many of the questions asked in this section. In a community and school setting, do you think supervision should be mandatory? Should you get paid as a supervisor? As a counselor? _____

_____

_____

_____

_____

DVD Transcripts from Group Supervision

TED: Hi, my name is Ted Chapin, I am a licensed psychologist and licensed marriage and family therapist, and today we are going to demonstrate group supervision for you. I would like to introduce our group today; maybe we could all go around and share our background and counseling, and then we could talk about some cases. Lori, would you like to start?

LORI: My name is Dr. Lori Russell-Chapin, I work full-time at Bradley University in Peoria, Illinois, and I work part-time for Chapin-Russell Associates, and I have been doing counseling for about 26 years now, and am really looking forward to being supervised today.

TED: Good.

BARBARA: My name is Barbara Peters, I work with Chapin-Russell, for 9 years now. I am a licensed clinical professional counselor, a licensed independent substance abuse counselor, recently got a certification in gerontology, and have been doing this for 23 years.

BRAD: My name is Brad Post, and I am a licensed clinical social worker and certified alcohol and drug abuse counselor, and I have been counseling for about 27 years, and I have specialties in addictions and anxiety disorders.

LISA: I am Lisa Rutherford, and I have been doing counseling for about 21 years, I think, and I have been at Chapin-Russell for 3 years. I have a master's in social work; I am a licensed clinical social worker; and I have specialties using EMDR, addictions, and anxiety disorders.

DEB: My name is Deb Kapitco, and I've got my master's in counseling, I am a nationally certified counselor, a licensed clinical professional counselor, I am also certified in EMDR, I am a trauma specialist and do a broad spectrum from sexual trauma to auto accidents. I have been doing this for about 8 years now.

JULIE: My name is Julie Roth. I am a recent graduate from Bradley University. I have my master's of arts in human development counseling, and since I am a novice, I am a generalist and have not specialized in anything as of yet.

TED: Okay, well it's great to have you all here today. We have a wide range of experience and backgrounds, and I hope we have a productive supervision session. One of the things we do to begin every session is just kind of get at the lay of the land, find out what kind of cases people are dealing with and would like some help with, so let's kind of talk about that first, if we can. What are some cases you would like some help with today?

LORI: Well, I have one.

TED: Lori, could you tell us a little bit about it?

LORI: I will be brief. This is a client I have seen off and on for 4 years, entered counseling for grief counseling. He lost both of his parents in a tragic accident and was just entering as a freshman in college, and every once in a while comes back because he goes away to college, and then he comes back, and some of his symptoms have changed, and he has now re-entered therapy because his girlfriend has just exited out of the picture.

TED: Okay.

LORI: And I just need some help.

TED: Help with grief counseling primarily then?

LORI: Uh-huh—well, grief counseling and then there is an added piece to it, so I have two supervision questions I'll ask you later.

TED: Okay. Others?

BRAD: I currently am working with a 15-year-old adolescent who was referred to me by the court system. I previously worked with his family, and the issues with this client have to do with the early stages of substance abuse, but more importantly, complicated factors of blended family issues and family systems issues in regard to extensive family history of chemical dependency and others' overreaction to that—excessive control leading to kind of a hopelessness in this teenager.

TED: Okay, so beginning stages of alcoholism and blended family issues?

BRAD: Yeah, early stages of abuse rather than dependency.

TED: Alcohol abuse?

BRAD: Yeah.

TED: Okay, anybody else have any item they would like to be sure they talk about today?

LISA: I have kind of a complicated case; I don't know if we'll have time to get to it, but a 46-year-old woman, white female with complicated PTSD, treatment is continually moving forward, then it stops, she keeps disengaging. She's had a lot of borderline characteristics; she engages with a lot of professionals and kind of spins her wheel a lot, but she keeps coming back to Chapin-Russell to work on the trauma. The current symptom that we're struggling with is anxiety going towards agoraphobia, and we've had a couple sessions just on the phone most recently.

TED: Okay, so PTSD with a client who comes and then takes off from counseling for a while?

LISA: Right, she's probably engaged in counseling with me four times now.

TED: Okay, anybody else have an item they would like to make sure we talk about?

BARBARA: Not today.

TED: Well, Lori, I guess, why don't we start with you.

LORI: Sure.

TED: Can you tell us some more about your case?

LORI: Sure. I just sort of have a case presentation guide, and I'll just go over it really quickly with you.

TED: Okay.

LORI: Again, I am going to call this person Sam—it's not his name—but he came in over his grief of his parents' death, and it was really sad because he just graduated from high school and he was on his way to go away to college, and so I began seeing him, and my history was I had seen his mother. I had never met this young man until I went to her funeral, and so presently he is a 23-year-old male, he is Caucasian, he has two siblings, uh . . . two sisters, and one brother. My client is the youngest; he is now graduated from college and has entered grad school. I think one of the reasons he has come back into therapy now was he has sort of been doing okay as he had been involved with this relationship, and she broke up with him, and as I was kind of getting him into some goals for counseling, I started getting into "What kind of coping skills do you have?" and he started telling me that he had a lot of anxiety and was using marijuana a lot, and when I say "a lot," on a daily basis most of the time. So my counseling goals were really to go over some—again grief issues because it felt to me like what was happening now was this grief was hitting him again, he really hadn't—he had done some grieving, but he hadn't got completely through with it, and now this was just hitting him over the head again with it. So I wanted to teach him some anxiety skills, some coping skills, and when we got into his marijuana use—I guess that is my supervision question. I wrote down, "How do I assist Sam in seeking treatment for daily pot addiction?" He gave it up for 10 days, that's the most he gave it in—I guess in evidently 2 years, and then when the girlfriend did not come back, he said, "I have to have it, this is my best friend, and you can't ask me to give up my best friend."

LISA: So that was a major issue in the relationship?

LORI: You know, Lisa, I really think it was, because as I dug into it, the girlfriend was saying, "I don't like this usage; I need you to stop that," and he really tried, but he doesn't have the skills to do it on his own. So that is my one supervision question, and the other one is—it's more personal—is, how do I ensure that I don't overstep my boundaries? We talk a lot about a therapeutic mom, but this kid, I just have to watch myself because what I want to do is take him home—I don't ever take him home, but I just want to take him home and feed him, and convince . . .

DEB: You want to mother him.

LORI: . . . I do, and so I think I do a really good job with boundaries therapy-wise, but I have this thing in me that's like, "Okay, I'll just—I can make him better," and so I have those two issues. I can tell you very quickly my DSM-IV-TR diagnosis. I gave him a V code of 62.82, which was bereavement, so we are working on that. I now have 304.30, which is cannabis dependence, and I also put down abuse; I think it's cannabis abuse.

There is deferred diagnosis on personality, AXIS II, no medical concerns that I can find at this point. He is exercising, he is starting to eat better, and I am getting him to exercise, which is good. I would say AXIS IV, my V codes are spiritual concerns, and I also wrote down, I think there are relational concerns with siblings; they're struggling with that. My GAF score Global Assessment of Functioning was about 65; I think there are some mild symptoms and some mild social difficulties.

TED: Okay, well, let's talk about . . .

LORI: (Sigh) I know that's how I feel like—(sigh).

TED: . . . Mom.

LORI: Mom?

TED: Yeah.

LORI: Talk about mom.

TED: Yeah, the feeling.

LORI: My mom?

TED: No—well, if you want to.

LORI: No, I don't want to talk about my mom. You mean my therapeutic mom?

TED: Yeah.

LORI: I really think I have been able to kind of keep my limits with him. A couple weeks ago when I saw Sam, he came in—I had not seen him—sometimes he does call me too on the phone because he goes away to college—I hadn't seen him in a while, he was disheveled, his hair was really long. I felt my mom—what I tell my children: cut your hair, take a bath, and, you know, those are the kinds of things I would want to say to my son, and so I sort of got into that. He said, "Well, it's just this casual look," and you know, he was disheveled, and at that point, I have to tell you—I can't tell you this is right, but at some point I said, "You know, Sam, if you were my son, let me tell you what I would say. I would tell you to cut your hair, I would tell you to take a bath, and I would tell you to get some lunch (because he hadn't eaten in a while), and I would tell you, then as your therapist, to get some treatment for marijuana abuse." And you know, we do have a decent relationship, so I mean I guess that is my response.

TED: What worries you about those feelings?

LORI: That I have to be careful about mom?

TED: Yeah.

LORI: I don't want to overstep my boundaries, and to me it's complicated because my real client was his mom. And so, he knew of me because I had met him at the funeral, and he said, "You know, I think my mother went to see you in therapy," and I didn't know what to say at that point, and so he started coming to see me. I think it's complicated for me because it's like I want to do the best I can for her because she's dead. I think I'm complicated with my own issues of mothering—so am I answering your question at all?

BRAD: Do you think he wants to be mothered, at this point? How is he responding to that kind of attention?

LORI: Oh, I think unconsciously he would love to be mothered, Brad. I think he would love to have someone take care of him, and you know he's lost. He's 23 years old and he does not have anybody in his life, and his brothers and sisters are married. Then when the girlfriend got rid of him, it was like—oh boy.

DEB: And he's using pot to survive and numb himself.

BRAD: Do you have enough of a relationship so far to be a mother with tough love?

LORI: Yes, I think I do, Brad, and I guess that is where I get confused. Where do I stop—you know, where do I go next? I have said to him, "You need to stop smoking marijuana," and one of the things, one of the strengths I have with Sam is that he is really intellectual, and so he is going to be a great attorney, actually, because he likes to fight—he loves to do that. And so what I try to do with him is, I make him get the facts. So he would say, "There is nothing wrong with the kind of marijuana that I use." So I would say, "Yeah, there is something wrong with it."

DEB: The kind.

LORI: Yeah, exactly. So I said, "Go research this for me," and he came back and he researched it, and he said, "Okay, the research says this," you know? And he realizes on a cognitive level how important that is, but I think on a heart level and a physiological level, he can't quit.

LISA: Did you review and identify the symptoms for him—the symptoms of addiction you see?

LORI: Yes, I have done that, so he's becoming aware that this is not helpful. The biggest thing—and you mentioned it, Lisa—was when he said, "Do you really think that this was one of the reasons that my girlfriend got rid of me?"

LISA: Uh-huh.

LORI: And I said yes, because I don't think he can be intimate when he's smoking pot like that.

BRAD: I think that . . . I think there are a lot of complicated factors to this. I think he is going to need more than just being asked to quit, obviously, if he's already gone back to it after such a short period of time. Um, I think you're on track by knowing he doesn't have the resources to succeed at that.

LORI: Uh-huh.

BRAD: So, I think making it your treatment goal for him to quit would be setting him up. I think it might be more wise to stay in that mother role, use it strategically . . .

LORI: Uh-huh.

BRAD: . . . and get him connected to the resources that can help him with that particular problem, but do that the way a mother would: educate him, do more research on your own. Provide him pictures of brain scans regarding the effects of marijuana—

LORI: That's good.

BRAD: —on his brain, but share . . .

BARBARA: Uh-huh, we have that.

BRAD: . . . rather than share it as a confronter, share it as an empathic person concerned about his well-being.

LORI: Comforting, kind of.

BRAD: Connect to him and continue building that relationship with him.

LORI: Well, I heard two things Brad. I thought—you know, I loved the idea of helping him, educate him, but I also thought I heard you say something about resources, that I could go and research, get the research and give him ideas about where he might want to go and present it that way.

LISA: Brain scans are a powerful visual thing.

BRAD: I have access to those.

LORI: Do you?

BRAD: So I can make you copies.

LORI: Oh, that would be so cool.

BRAD: I can print them out for you.

LORI: That would be so good, that would be so good.

DEB: And that's counterproductive of his goal. He wants to be a lawyer, I thought you said?

LORI: Uh-huh.

DEB: Okay, so he's affecting his brain right now.

LISA: He's compromising his success—that's a motivator.

LORI: Absolutely.

LISA: I have one question, Lori.

LORI: Uh-huh.

LISA: Did he use marijuana before his parents were killed?

LORI: No.

LISA: Okay, so he would have to learn to deal with emotions and process through that probably, and start over with grief and help him process through those emotions and what he is not doing. He needs to learn again how to not deal with—how to deal with life without using.

LORI: Uh-huh.

LISA: Because he hasn't for 2 years.

LORI: Uh-huh.

LISA: So, I kind of agree with Brad; to say "just stop," without dealing with those emotions and the fear and what's going on with him and that level, he's going to struggle to not use marijuana.

DEB: He's got to replace it with something.

LORI: Absolutely.

LISA: Right.

BRAD: The other complicating factor here, ultimately, with that frequency of use is, it basically completely dampers the part of the brain that creates motivation for change, so the discomfort of his grief, the discomfort of what he's doing to himself, the feedback for that is missing.

LORI: Yeah.

BRAD: As a result of him using every single day, the midbrain section, the part of the brain that manages his emotional response—you know, the energy of his emotions it creates movement for—isn't accessed; he isn't feeling it.

LORI: Uh-huh.

BRAD: And, um, he might not even feel your confrontation or concern in a true deep sense as long as he's using like that. And again, these are things you have to educate him with and let him know that he's actually stifling his experience, even your relationship with him—that result—to continue to use and—um, building a relationship with him is going to be difficult as long he's using every day. Its almost a catch-22; you can only get in so far and make such a connection with him because his marijuana use isn't going to allow him to actually experience the relationship.

LORI: Well—and I think, Brad, that the advantage I've had is that I had a relationship with him before that, so I had that rapport. The other thing I have is that connection to his mother.

BRAD: And that's what I said; I would go back to taking advantage of that surrogate mother role if he values that and is looking for it; use it strategically as a way to create motivation, because if you've already had that relationship, he's going to be tapping into that external motivation more than he is going to be tapping into his own resources because he's not going to feel it.

LISA: So, you are saying, Lori, that you could use your knowledge of his mother.

LORI: And I have.

LISA: And tap into some of her values on intimacy and relationships and what he's missing now as a result of the marijuana use.

LORI: I think I could do that.

LISA: And the ending of the relationship—great peace could come of that very easily.

LORI: I think I could do that. Absolutely.

DEB: Alright, now how motivated is he to stop smoking pot? It's pretty limited isn't it?

LORI: I think it depends on the day, I mean, I think there are some days where he says, "I know this is not good for me and I want to do it differently," and then there are some days where he says, "Forget it," you know?

LISA: The emotions come up.

LORI: Uh-huh.

DEB: Does he get high when he comes in to see you?

LORI: No, that's very interesting, that's the one thing I have—I have set up boundaries that you may not do that, and only one time have I asked him to leave.

BRAD: He is able to regulate the time of day then, but not his use from day to day.

LORI: Yeah.

BRAD: The catch-22 with this again is, you know, can he connect, you know, to the relationship side of this? But, um, I've done it with clients who have been using marijuana daily, where I've tried to build the relationship to see if it would evolve into a greater motivation as a result of the relationship. When you get into daily use, procrastination becomes the primary response: you know, "I'll get to that," or I'm going to," or—um, so at some place you may appoint a time—you may be forced to set a boundary regarding continuing counseling—

LORI: That's great; I was wondering about that.

BRAD: —with you, if he chooses not to consider doing it at all.

TED: Could you be more specific, Brad—like how you might go about setting that kind of boundary?

BRAD: Well, I think the first part is to make sure you give him all the information regarding what you know to be the apparent effects of this drug, in terms of ability to benefit his therapy process and deal with his grief, and let him know that you are going to expect him to open himself up to the idea of problem solving as part of your relationship with him—that you can talk about problem solving and coming up with coping techniques that he could use to deal with his grief more effectively as an alternative to using marijuana, and see if he can actually incorporate some of those, because if he has some additional resources to be able to problem solve and he can demonstrate he can actually apply those, then maybe he can find a way to be more motivated to let go if he has something to replace it with. But if he starts bargaining with you or making excuses or talking about why he is not doing it this week and that goes on for two or three sessions, then, you know, I think you probably need to be a little more emphatic with a tough love side in terms of your concern about the ongoing relationship being beneficial to him therapeutically, if he continues to use marijuana or doesn't seek out help to break the cycle of that. I even give clients—I bargain with them to teach them more about their addiction: "If you don't want to see a therapist or see a specialist to deal with your addiction, will you set that as a personal goal and work on that on your own right now?" as a way to actually give them experience of not being able to stop, and then use that as another intervention. "You said you were going to work on this, to cut back. You weren't able to do that; this is a pretty strong sign you have developed an addiction, and you may need more assistance," so you know allow him the opportunity to fail, but add it into the treatment plan goal with you—

LORI: I think that's great.

BRAD: —so you can use it as a feedback loop.

LORI: That would be a great idea.

BRAD: Let him bargain with you if he chooses to, in the grief process of giving up his marijuana, but then give him feedback about how he's doing that.

LORI: Uh-huh, that sounds excellent.

DEB: So then marijuana came on with the death of his parents?

LORI: Yes, gradually it came on with the death.

DEB: But he found that skill to compensate for not feeling, to shut down the grief.

LORI: Uh-huh, absolutely, I really think that's what it was; I mean he knows that this is his best friend right now, unfortunately.

BRAD: Are you sure he did not use it at all before, or did not use as often?

LORI: He did not use it in high school.

BRAD: Okay.

LORI: And the summer that he was going to college, his parents got killed.

BARBARA: The summer before he started.

LORI: Yes.

DEB: And were his parents killed in an auto accident, or just . . .

LORI: A plane crash.

DEB: Oh, so you're looking at the trauma—

LORI: Absolutely.

DEB: —a major trauma link there as well, 'cause trauma and the addiction goes hand in hand, so EMDR could be beneficial for him, to even help. If the trauma is feeding him and he needs to desensitize himself with, you know, the mood-altering substances, first its being able to desensitize it with the EMDR and work though that trauma piece. Once working through that trauma piece, then they can engage in treatment more effectively. When I was at a substance abuse treatment facility working with women that were sexually abused, going in and doing EMDR on their sexual trauma allowed them to engage in their treatment, and before that they were just re-acting out their trauma all the time.

LORI: Sure that's a good idea too; I've got some great ideas.

TED: Lori, I want to go back, if I can, to the problem side of the mother feelings in the relationship.

LORI: Well, I knew you would.

TED: Can you give us some examples where those come up, where you begin to feel uncomfortable or uncertain as to its impact?

LORI: Um, recently, Mothers' Day—just that whole feeling of, you know, I tried to encourage Sam to acknowledge the fact it was Mother's Day and to do something constructive for his mother, visit her grave, do something, but my immediate feeling was "Okay, you can come to my house for dinner; we're having a really nice Mothers' Day." I'd never—I have never done that, but that is that feeling I have, it's like ooh.

LISA: But you wanted to.

LORI: I do, and the part I didn't tell, you when I told him to get his hair cut, he went and got his hair cut—he just looked so darling—I mean, he looked so like a nice good kid.

BRAD: That's what I was wondering, whether or not he was actually looking for—because if he is, again you might be able to use that as a motivational piece for him in terms of working through the intervention with the marijuana stuff and seeking out assistance with that. He may be looking for somebody to . . .

LORI: I think he might be.

BRAD: . . . guide him that way.

LORI: And I think that tough love piece.

BRAD: His resistance might not be very strong if—there may be more fear than resistance.

TED: But what might be the downside?

BRAD: If she looked into it too much.

TED: If you were stuck in that kind of feeling, what might be the downside of assuming that?

LISA: It would be harder to confront.

TED: Harder to confront.

LISA: Uh-huh, it would be harder maybe. It would be easy, I think, for some people to fall into what mothers do: minimizing, denying issues, or problems that are coming up and calling it something else—mothers do that for their children.

LORI: That's interesting, Lisa, because I think that's the downside of my being a mother is I don't minimize. With our kids I think I make it too big.

DEB: Maximize.

LORI: I think I do, and so I try to make sure I am not doing that, but I think it's this tough love piece, this is what I would do with my son. This is probably what I need to do with Sam.

BRAD: For him, though, it may—I mean, I think the danger in his recovery would be that he replaces his mom with you instead of deal with the real loss of his mother.

JULIE: Escaping.

LORI: Yeah.

DEB: The expectation of you rescuing and saving him, then set you up as "well, because if I don't succeed with him, then am I failing?"

LORI: Sure. Well, the neat thing about this relationship is that we have talked about, you know, "I am not your mother, I can never be your mother, and I don't want to be your mother, you don't want me to be your mother." We've had that conversation in counseling, so I am really happy about that.

BRAD: At least it's on the table now, you can watch for it in an emergency.

LORI: Yeah, absolutely.

TED: I guess I wonder if those needs that he has for being nurtured—somehow, if there are other ways that he can be encouraged to meet those needs in his life. You mentioned relationships with siblings is an issue. Could you say more about that and maybe the thought of are there other areas of sources of support for him too?

LORI: Well, see, I think his siblings are a source of support, but they're also lost too, you know—they're also lost, they lost their parents too. Now they have been recently married and those kinds of things, but I think the piece that might need to be replaced is the piece of spirituality and trying to get him back into his own spirituality. I think that would be a resource, but he doesn't want to go there because it reminds him of his childhood, because they were very strong.

JULIE: Does he talk with his siblings?

LORI: Oh, absolutely.

JULIE: I mean about the memories.

LORI: Yes, yes, he does and that is a very nice thing—they do talk about it—but I think another thing, he's struggling; he's the youngest now and everybody wants to tell him what to do.

JULIE: Right.

LORI: And I think that is another piece that he's struggling with.

DEB: Well, you mentioned one of your goals is for spirituality; has he like turned against God because he took his parents away?

LORI: I don't know if he's turned against it; he's confused. I don't think he's turned against it; he's confused with it, and we've worked a lot on that issue trying to get him to test the waters—you know, "Have you thought about going back to church, go to different kinds of churches?"

BARBARA: Try something new.

LORI: Yeah, absolutely, so he's thinking about it.

LISA: EMDR can help with that too.

LORI: Okay.

LISA: The trauma link to that block right now.

LORI: I like that, those are great.

LISA: EMDR helps with that often.

LORI: Okay, that's wonderful.

DEB: Does he ever talk about the accident, or is it complete . . .

LORI: Oh yeah, we talk about it.

DEB: . . . so he will move towards it.

LORI: Yeah.

DEB: And is he hyperaroused when he moves towards it?

LORI: Sometimes.

DEB: Like even assessing, when you think about that picture, when you found out that your parents had died in the plane crash, what comes up for you? And 0–10, how disturbing is that to—you know, how much is it processed?

LORI: I think he has worked on some of that, but I still think it wouldn't be a bad idea to see if we could get him through some of those pieces.

TED: Any other thoughts for Lori?

LORI: Well, I appreciate this because I think you've answered my supervision questions. I love the brain scan pictures, I really like this idea of tough love and the mothering, the EMDR, and even the EMDR with spirituality—I think that piece is really helpful, so I think you've helped a lot. Thank you. I'm ready to go.

TED: Let us know what happens.

LORI: Okay, I will thank you.

TED: Let's see, Brad—adolescent, blended family issues, maybe the beginnings of alcohol abuse.

BRAD: Yeah, this is a really complicated case from a systems standpoint, so I'll just kind of give you the background and then kind of go into my questions with this. I had worked with this boy's mother, off and on with her, addressing issues with his two older siblings, over a period of about 5 or 6 years, who have both developed alcohol and drug abuse problems or dependency problems. It's that relationship with this mother historically, but he was actually referred to me by a court advocate as a result of being arrested for alcohol—illegal consumption of alcohol—with his sister driving the vehicle as the older adult in the vehicle and supplying it to him and his friends, and she took off—basically evaded the police and left the state—took off with her boyfriend and is now on the lam, so to speak. There is a warrant out for her arrest because she stole the vehicle, and her boyfriend has a warrant out for his arrest, so it's very complicated on the legal side. This was my client's first arrest, and he's on what's called a second chance program for the court system, and being monitored by the school advocate. His parents divorced when he was young, only 2 or 3. His natural father is alcohol dependent, untreated, he has two half-siblings from his father's first marriage, who are both alcoholic and drug addicted, and his two older siblings are alcohol and drug dependent. His brother went through this process of the system the same that way he did, and ended up running away from the police and violating probation and is now on the lam in another state in another part of the country. So he has seen all of this kind of unfold ahead of him, and he's been "a good child"—

JULIE: Right.

BRAD: —up until the last year and a half. He's begun to experiment, but he's a lost child as well, and his mother's preoccupation kind of focuses on helping deal with his older brother's situation and his sister's situation—kind of left him in the background. His relationship with this stepfather is kind of neutral—not much of a relationship and no antagonism or negative energy. His family is fairly well-to-do and so one of the benefits of being in this family system is they travel all around the world together and go on all kinds of adventures together in the summer, but during the school year things are very tense. His mother's response to having a third child get involved in substance abuse has been to completely clamp down on him and restrict everything. She's put in hidden cameras, basically has surveillance on him 24 hours a day. She's moved him out of his own bedroom into a supervised area of the house into his sister's old room—it's decorated in pink—and taken the doors off of the bedroom door and has hidden cameras all over the place. He will be in certain places—like he'll be sitting in his classroom at school, and he'll see her drive by and slow down and look in the room. When he finally earns privileges to be off restriction, she's usually there within 5 minutes and he sees her circling, wherever he's at, in the car to watch where he's at.

TED: What is his reaction to all that?

BRAD: He has no relationship with this mother, there's zero respect, completely alienated from her. I don't think they really had a relationship before this problem unfolded recently—this happened earlier in the year—and so I think the ground for this kind of unraveled and the groundwork for this unraveling was already set up.

JULIE: Is he aware of the hidden cameras?

BRAD: Oh yeah, he's the one that's told me about them.

JULIE: Okay.

BRAD: I just confront it with the mother, and she said, "Oh yeah, these are the things that I've done." She actually found out that from a rumor that they were driving together, and she called the police to have them arrested, and so she set it up so that a consequence would occur to hold them accountable, which is what she did with her son to get him the treatment originally. It was actually successful to get him in the treatment because it was court mandated because she tried on her own to get him to cooperate with treatment and he never did. But he is now required to go through counseling; he signed the contract to go through counseling and was referred to me. I carefully evaluated whether or not his seeing me was an issue since his mother had seen me, and he really doesn't have an issue with that. We were able to build rapport fairly quickly by me simply empathizing with his experience with all the excessive control and the dynamics of his family system. And so it's moving along in that direction. Basically, the goals for counseling for his mother are for him to achieve abstinence, to educate him about chemical dependency and help him establish a plan to prevent this from unraveling like it has for his siblings and his extended family, to help him prove his communication with his mother and clarify his goals for visitation because there is a complicating factor in this, which is that his personal goal is to get out of the home with his mother and move in with his natural father. His natural father is the busy kind of dad type of person; his dad is a golfer, and that's a strong interest of his. And so his mom has full custody; his dad has no actual rights to any kind of direction to his upbringing, but he does have visitation. So his father really doesn't have the right to take him to his home, and he keeps telling his son, kind of building him up that he's going to do something to get custody of him. He's a 15-year-old; however, his father doesn't not have the financial resources to follow through with it and make it happen, so he's building his son up and triangulating him against his mother in the process. The more that happens, the more crazy mom gets, the more she clamps down, the more resistive she becomes to my ideas of giving him an opportunity to build trust, and again there's no work taking place in the relationship. His personal goal is to get through the court process and get them off of his back and move in with his father. I think he is compliant with substance abuse treatment right now, but I don't think he is internally motivated. He doesn't meet the criteria for dependence yet: alcohol abuse, he reports 10–12 times of drinking; cannabis, he reports maybe 15–16 times of use since he started, going back to seventh grade.

LISA: Do you still see the mom too?

BRAD: Mother was recently in treatment with another therapist and dropped out of therapy when that person confronted her about why she had her son arrested. She lost faith in that person and ended therapy with that person, so she's currently not in individual counseling herself.

TED: What are your questions for supervision for us?

BRAD: I need help coming up with some strategies for engaging mother's trust for the process of loosening up the reins a little bit. I do not see this succeeding at all if she remains in 24-hour surveillance of her son. He needs to be given a chance to succeed, and he doesn't have any hope at all. After five sessions, he still kind of—in my kind of convincing him that I would advocate for him in this process, he does not believe that it will make any difference at all. I'm trying to work with him at trying to come up with something to get me to negotiate with, so to speak, with his mother.

TED: He's just wanting out.

BRAD: He's wanting out and he doesn't have an out; it's really not an option.

DEB: This is his second chance and be done with that then.

BRAD: I'm concerned that he's going to sabotage this.

DEB: Yeah.

BRAD: And basically set himself up for failure because he didn't see any hope, really any hope in it being different. So I am looking for some, maybe some ideas that maybe I haven't thought of to strategically help mom let go and focus more on the relationship with him. There's a couple of ways—there's a couple of things that are in place right now that might help with that. One is that the court monitor—the court advocate is responsible for monitoring his compliance with all these things, so I would let him be the bad guy and her move into focusing on the relationship issues.

DEB: So would they drop him and . . .

BRAD: They are dropping him and monitoring and checking with him weekly at school and all those things.

LORI: Let me ask—so as I listen to you talk—so mom basically, according to son, is just pretty pig-headed, stubborn, is not going to let go of anything, and is just holding on as tightly as she can, but there is no relationship.

BRAD: He doesn't have any respect or desire for a relationship with her, doesn't really believe she has one other than to control him.

JULIE: And was that prior to his use?

BRAD: Prior to his arrest with this particular situation that occurred earlier in the year, but he had been caught with marijuana use, or she would have read his e-mails previously discussing experimentation with marijuana use, and she started clamping on down back then.

JULIE: So she really didn't have a lot of trust in him even before the arrest or—with two children prior using.

BRAD: Both who have left the state because of her control issues, ultimately.

DEB: And are these the same dynamics—she's always been this controlling person, despite the fact—

BRAD: She went from being an enabler . . .

DEB: Okay, that's what it is.

BRAD: . . . and being codependent with her children and really not focusing on preventing this and educating about the process—when they first got into trouble—coming in to help. With me, we began to set boundaries and are doing it fairly constructively, not with overkill, you know—setting boundaries, doing progressive discipline, following through with letting them make a mistake, and then holding them accountable and giving all that information to them ahead of time, so they're given choices ahead of time. With him, her response has been just absolute protection, control, "I'm not going to let you mess up again."

LISA: So coming from that perspective, a lot of what she's doing is a trauma response to the failure with her two older ones, so to get her reengaged in counseling to try to help her so she is validated—you know, "I'm being kind of a victim of life"—to get her in, you can join with her there. Yes, you have had a hard time, you deserve help and coming from the point of trauma because of the hypervigilance. I mean, you have identified several symptoms of PTSD that gets in her way of being able to become less rigid.

BRAD: It's multigenerational for her, the trauma is not just with her children, it's with her ex-husbands, and with her family of origin. It's been repeated out in one generation after another.

LISA: So she sees no other option until, you know, that gets treated to become less rigid—it's not safe.

BRAD: Well, and the counselor that she was working with, who was trying to move her into becoming to become less rigid, she fired.

LISA: But you can't do that before treating the trauma. I think that's the key piece. She doesn't know what else to do.

LORI: It seems to me the word we haven't used today is fear. Mom is just so afraid.

BRAD: Oh, she's terrified. This is all based on fear.

DEB: There he goes down the same road.

TED: Well, I'm wondering about anger too. Anger that's sort of focused and projected onto the kid, for who knows all of what.

BRAD: I think these screw-ups for each of these children may have actually been pre-destined by that anger.

LISA: And her trauma.

DEB: Well, he's the only one she can get to now.

BRAD: Right.

LORI: Yeah.

BRAD: Right.

LORI: If you ask, and you have—I'm sure you've asked this question—but what's the biggest thing she's most afraid of? What would she say?

BRAD: I think before this happened, it would be for him to get involved in the same path that his brother and sister have had and that he becomes an addict. I think at this point in time it's that she is going to lose her son.

LORI: And she can't see the paradox that with what she's doing, she is going to lose her son.

BRAD: (Shakes head yes)

LORI: She can't see that yet. You've said that to her?

BRAD: Yes, and she's had other counselors tell her the same thing. She has the court advocate telling her that, and she also has the other counselor that she sees.

DEB: So she's creating what she fears.

BRAD: And she's afraid of most of it being played out. And she's really not functioning—well, she's deteriorating significantly. I think she has major depression and is just barely getting by.

TED: What are his resources? How is he doing in school, his social system?

BRAD: He's a bright student, he has relationships, although not with people that she is in favor of. All of his friends are under suspension.

TED: Are they worthy of suspension?

BRAD: Some of them are, some of them clearly are. I mean the point—the validation of her experience in every step of the way is that she's not delusional. I mean this is stuff that is really happening right out in front of her. You know, in terms of the severity of these choices and the people he's choosing to hang with, he's probably higher—out of the group of people he hangs with—he's probably the highest functioning of the group.

TED: But he's doing well in school?

BRAD: He's doing average to above average

TED: Okay, interests, activities?

BRAD: Sports and golf primarily.

LORI: She can't follow him around the golf course can she?

BRAD: She does.

LORI: Oh my stars!

DEB: She's got a camera in the cart.

BRAD: She follows—I think she follows his father and him around.

DEB: Yeah—have you met with dad at all?

BRAD: Dad has been semiresistant to participating. He'll have conversations on the phone, but he's reluctant to participate and often makes promises that he doesn't keep.

DEB: There's a concern that dad's really setting him up.

BRAD: (Shakes head yes)

DEB: You know he's setting a goal, but it's not going to happen.

BRAD: My issue with that process is dad has no legal rights or custody issues, and mom refuses to allow him to participate. She lets me talk to him on the phone just to clarify how things are going over there.

TED: Is the dad in any way a positive resource for him?

BRAD: I think dad's part of—I mean dad feeds, naturally, his chemistry into the triangulation, actually undermines and minimizes all of this.

TED: I mean do they share a golf interest, for example, Brad?

BRAD: The son and his father? Oh, he has high respect for his father. That's his only relationship, and he's overly attached to his father, and he's got him on a pedestal, despite his father's low functioning and his father's poor choices and handling of his relationship with his mother.

DEB: And you say the father's—

BRAD: And I don't even know if he's involved in promoting the substance abuse from the alcohol use. I don't think my client would tell me that if he was.

TED: What does the son feel about his situation, this kid?

BRAD: Hopeless.

TED: He feels hopeless.

BRAD: He feels trapped, he feels like he doesn't have any options. He moves to fantasy problem solving or magical thinking about his father rescuing him from this and taking him out of the home.

JULIE: And did your client have a desire to be with his father full-time even before his use and getting into trouble.

BRAD: Before getting in trouble the first time . . .

JULIE: Right.

BRAD: . . . or when he first got caught with the drugs. I would say for the last year and a half, 2 years, he's been interested in going with his father.

JULIE: I guess I'm wondering if this is perhaps your client's way, one of the ways, he's had models that, you know, got out of the state. Could this be a way for him to get to his father: if he messes up enough with his mom, maybe his mom will just give up, where he can leave town like his siblings?

LORI: So he's doing what? That's all he knows, right? This worked for his sister.

BARBARA: Any suicidal ideation on his part?

BRAD: No, no self-abuse, no self-harm, no suicidal issues, nothing on any—you know turning it inward onto himself. His anger's directed mostly at his mom and it's polarized by the response that she has in terms of control. It's tempered itself quite a bit since he's been on court supervision in March because that feedback loop is now involved in the legal process, and there is potential in him having more severe consequences if he follows the process out the way his brother and sister did. He sees his sister's situation interestingly—since his sister's on the lam, he sees his sister's situation as being self-defeating, but he sees his brother's situation as being kind of admirable; he got out, now he's got a job and is living on his own in Florida, and things are better.

DEB: But that was after he was on the lam.

BRAD: He went through the whole process, though; his brother only had like 4 months to go to complete the whole process.

TED: Maybe that is the path to independence for this family, unfortunately.

DEB: He is a criminal.

TED: And normally I am the family systems advocate, but I am hearing so many roadblocks in the family system to intervene with this kid. I find myself more wondering about how to build the resources for this kid, or build on the resources he does have, how to help him learn how to . . .

BRAD: Become independent.

TED: . . . through these choices and make decisions and see consequences and make choices that hopefully are to his advantage in his life, in his personal life, whatever he can control it.

BRAD: That's one of the things we talked about in terms of clarifying his goal for therapy, whether or not he wants to work on a relationship with family or to work on his own issues, but when we talk about it in that perspective, for him—3 years until he is independent at 18 is a lifetime to him. It's like it might as well be 100 years. Dealing with his mother for 3 more years is beyond his comprehension.

TED: Yeah.

BRAD: One of the things I tried to do is to hook him into some other things. The golf thing he has a really—a problem, a real bad swing right now, and he keeps shanking the ball, and he talks about it every session, so we got into some sports psychology stuff and some imagery; and the last week, using the imagery work I have been dealing with him, he's actually got his ball to start going straight down the fairway. So I'm hooking into some other things in our relationship building with him to try to help with focusing on that, and so I think if I stay in that direction I'll be okay with him as long as he's court mandated to be involved in counseling with me. I think we can continue building a relationship, and maybe that will go a little bit further. But I really see this being temporary if the family systems stuff doesn't lighten up a little bit. There's kind of a catch-22 here.

LORI: You're less concerned about the son, but you seem to be more concerned about mom. Are you going to try to get her back into counseling?

BRAD: I am concerned about mom sabotaging what I am accomplishing with her son.

LORI: Are going to try to get her into counseling then?

BRAD: I plan to talk to her again about—if not going back and working out the differences she had with the previous counselor, to consider referral from me to someone else.

JULIE: Well, and I think you were alluding to this, but when you were working with the sports psychology, the golf, and how going back to when he was so disappointed and he was shanking the ball—and could he relate to being hopeless in that sense?

BRAD: Oh yeah.

JULIE: I am never going to fix this.

BRAD: He in fact quit golfing for 2 weeks.

JULIE: Yeah, but then, make it parallel: you know, he's now straightened out his—how can we, you know, bring that over to his life? And this hopeless situation, how can you, you know, straighten out that?

LORI: Because you had control over that.

JULIE: Exactly.

BARBARA: You mentioned that he has gotten more compliant since he's been since March and he sees the consequences of this system.

BRAD: After being on house arrest for 2 months.

BARBARA: Yeah, so he's intelligent enough to see the consequences, and he's—you could call it working the system, but he's getting better.

BRAD: He's getting better, but he's not really getting any kind of real payoff for it, and I'm afraid that if the payoff doesn't come soon, he's going to go back into that kind of hopeless framework, because he finally earned his curfew leaving the house and being home by 5:00 p.m., and like I said, he was being monitored by his mother, and she—the first day he was out, he saw her seven times within 35 minutes.

LORI: That's amazing!

JULIE: See, she's not rewarding—when he's gaining something like curfew, she's not letting go at that point.

BRAD: What she perceives as a reward is not really a reward.

JULIE: Right, so she's not, you know, letting up, even when he gains.

BRAD: They're not agreeing on the reward definitions.

JULIE: Exactly.

TED: Is she refusing then to reward him?

BRAD: She said she's considering what I suggest, and then when I get feedback from him the next session, she's not doing it.

TED: So I am wondering if you could do some reframing somehow of his failure as really being good events, good successes for him to understand the boundaries and limits, and the more that happens outside of her, the better for him to learn about how to be responsible for his own choices, and maybe you can reframe somehow the successes, since her mindset is to minimize those that—yeah, you're right; I mean to agree with her somehow that those aren't really as important as is his really learning how to do this himself, change the whole focus of this from compliance with her to sort of growth for him.

LISA: I think that imagery could help do that with the skills you mentioned earlier to help him to be able to—

TED: Like the golf metaphor?

LISA: —visualize how he can be successful in life.

TED: Yeah.

LISA: And how he can start doing that now.

LORI: Well, I see the golf's really nice too because—not that I know much about golf, but I think there are so many different skills that you do with each iron or each wood or, you know, you do with putting or to do a long shot. I think if we could somehow get him to get involved in that and then say, "Do you understand this is a skill you need as you get close to a hole?" and I think those might work with him.

BRAD: I might have to consult a golf pro or get assistance from one.

LORI: You might have to—really, Brad, that might not be a bad idea though.

JULIE: Yeah, I think it would attract because with golf—I mean, there's a sweet spot and you will spend 18 holes.

LORI: Are you a golfer, Julie?

JULIE: Yes, and it can be the worst game—you know, the worst 18 holes, and then you decide, okay, one more round, and then you hit the sweet spot, and it was worth it, and you keep going.

LISA: And the other shots leave your mind.

JULIE: Yes, exactly.

LORI: Variable schedule of reinforcement right there.

JULIE: Exactly.

LORI: Well, I think that's a great idea. I like the golf idea too. I think the sweet spot might be a neat thing to talk about—what is his sweet spot?

LISA: How does it feel?

LORI: Yeah, when you do hit the sweet spot, what's that like?

LISA: The work you do to get there.

LORI: Yeah, I like that. And you know, Brad, I, see now this is very nontraditional, but this would be something I know I would do: I'd take him out to a—like, a three-hole golf-thing course and have him teach you—have him teach you something. I think I would have him teach you about golf

LISA: Yeah, he could be your pro.

LORI: I think that would be so interesting, because how often does someone say to you, "You're an expert; you know what you're doing. I need to know more about the sweet spot." I mean do you even know about the woods and the irons?

BRAD: Oh yeah.

LORI: Well you could fake it then; you could pretend you don't know.

BRAD: The woods is where you hunt.

BARBARA: And the iron is what presses your clothes.

LORI: The iron is the little grid that you're in now in your mother's house—but I think that would be really interesting to take him to, like, a small golf course and have him—or hit a bucket of balls with him.

BRAD: Or to the driving range.

LORI: Yeah, I think that would be so neat.

LISA: Let him be the expert.

LORI: I like that. I think that would be really cool.

TED: And there's a definition of success that maybe mom can understand and disengage from because that's really his doing, his creating, not mom's overseeing.

DEB: And if she can allow the courts to take over, and like you said, make them be the bad guy because . . .

BRAD: She needs to build a relationship with her son. She's got to start from below ground zero.

JULIE: And how interesting, though, that's not anywhere in the goals, communication with the son and mother in that relationship, you know from her perspective.

DEB: I am not sure if she's capable.

TED: Maybe that's her therapy issue for herself. Maybe after doing some other work to be able to communicate in those relationships.

BRAD: Well, I mean the key issue in all this for me—I guess my last supervision question has to do with how to help them build trust with each other, because it's completely—it's been annihilated.

LISA: I think you need them to do that; for one thing, to get them to start working together as a team instead of opponents using this kid in the middle.

BRAD: It's not going to happen.

LISA: If he feels hopeless in being able to do that.

BRAD: It's not going to happen. They were in mediation in the court process for almost 11 years to try to work that out, and it's not going to happen.

LISA: But their son's the victim.

BRAD: Oh, I know, absolutely.

LORI: Well, I still go back to golf then. I still think in the trust issue—that how do you, when you golf—and Julie I'm taking this to you—when you golf, how did you learn to trust that you could use a 9 iron, or that you could use a 1 wood, or how did you learn to trust that?

JULIE: Well, one, it's getting over the fear of people watching you on the first tee.

LORI: Okay.

JULIE: And which iron . . .

LORI: Because they are watching, I actually think they are watching.

JULIE: Right, it's with the woods and the big bertha—and so then having that confidence to try it out, but then you have to use it.

LORI: You have to keep practicing.

JULIE: You have to keep doing it and, you know, seek out help and have someone watch you.

BRAD: Would you write down a list of all the slang terms?

LORI: I like the big bertha thing. But I think there's something about that, I think there's something that—that you could build trust that way, and I am convinced you are on the right track with mother too. I think mother has to deal with her issues and son, and maybe it's too late with son and mother, but it's not too late for son to have a life, and it's not too late for mother to have a life, but perhaps if they could—perhaps later down the road they could get together.

JULIE: And also some, like, bonding exercises, where they have to work as a team—and even if it's for 30 minutes in session—but where they have to communicate, they have to work together; otherwise, I mean, like Raccoon Circles is one that comes to mind, where they have to be a team, because right now they are not at all, and even if its for 30 minutes, or for 2 minutes, that's 2 minutes longer than . . .

LISA: Yeah, I would go more for 2.

JULIE: . . . that might be a start, a foot in the door.

LISA: Like a computer game or something.

JULIE: Yeah, there's also Raccoon Circles—that's what I'm familiar with—where there's like a rope, and there are exercises that they can do as a family—you know, 2 people up to 30—and it's just team building, where they have to like lean against each other, but balance, and so it's working together—otherwise one person will fall. And there's a myriad of exercises, and it's free online.

TED: I guess I find myself still wondering what might be good about the relationship with dad. There must be—I presume there's something good there, something that I would find to be encouraging of or support. I guess I am hearing mom say it's all bad.

BRAD: Oh, for me to convince mom of, you mean?

TED: No, not to convince mom of, but to help the kid connect to with his dad, the healthy part of his dad.

BRAD: He's already connected to his father, so I don't see that as an issue.

LORI: You're saying use . . .

TED: In a healthy way though, Brad.

BRAD: He chooses the discussion because it's open to interpretation, but for him . . .

TED: Maybe that's a theme of self-sufficiency or perseverance, or I don't know what that would be, but something he could grab a hold of there because he's identifying with dad it sounds like, and not with mom.

LISA: Loyalty.

DEB: But that's the fantasy and the escape right? "Oh, this could happen."

BRAD: I'm not—I mean, I don't even remember a session where dad has even come up between the client and me as a therapeutic issue in terms of resistance or interference or any of those things, because I've been very careful to kind of empathize with where he's at, so I don't think—I mean those conversations have taken place with mom and with the advocate, but not with the client. I don't think the client perceives me as having any negative views of his father in regard to that dynamic.

LORI: You know, the other thing, Brad, that makes me think of this trust issue you mentioned earlier was this whole piece of—you said it didn't take you long to build rapport with this young man.

BRAD: He has strong needs for attention, strong needs for connection.

LORI: And so—and it's a male identification as well. I wonder if you can help him continue to build trust, I mean if the relationship with mom is not going to get better.

TED: To learn to build trust.

LORI: Yeah, if that—I mean, I really think that happens in therapy, so if you could do that—and have you talked to him about your relationship with him?

BRAD: Not much.

LORI: I think that would be a really interesting piece because he doesn't have a lot of healthy role models, and I think, Brad, if you could share it with him, that might be a place to go.

BRAD: That's a real good idea.

LISA: But a significant piece—you know, again going back to what Ted is saying, you know, help him connect with these skills within himself, learning to trust his decisions, his coping—you know, staying true to what he believes, trusting himself.

TED: I guess one more thought about dad—I know I am beating—

DEB: I keep thinking about dad too.

BRAD: Father's Day is in 3 weeks.

TED: Maybe that's what it is, I don't know. I remember some cases, Brad, where the mom has sort of polarized against the dad, the kid is in the middle, and mom has had primary custody for years, and the kid has all these questions and fantasies and ideals of what dad is and what he would be like, and it's almost as though—to me, there's no way he's going to find out about that unless he gets a chance to have that experience with his dad.

BRAD: You misunderstood me. He does have a relationship with his father; he sees him twice a week.

TED: Okay.

BRAD: He sees him on Saturdays and Wednesdays.

LORI: Okay.

BRAD: He gets visitation with his dad, so they have contact, and they do things together.

TED: But I mean even for him to take that to the next step he wants to someday . . .

BRAD: Just have a relationship with dad and . . .

TED: . . . which might be living with dad and learning about dad as an ideal and learning about fantasy and reality, and facing those issues himself could be a good thing in the long run.

DEB: 'Cause why didn't he—why doesn't he have any legal rights? He just has supervision—I mean, he just has visitation.

BRAD: Because of his abuse to the client's mother, his alcohol abuse or dependency, he was basically found unfit by the court.

DEB: Okay.

TED: There's a lot of stuff there on both sides.

LISA: Dad's not the perfect role model either.

TED: No, no, but that's his family, his life.

BRAD: Believe it or not, this is the healthiest—this 15-year-old is the healthiest person in the system . . .

JULIE: It sounds like it.

BARBARA: Oh, yeah.

LORI: Yeah, I'm sure.

BRAD: . . . except for the stepfather, which he doesn't really have any kind of a bond with, other than . . .

BARBARA: Oh, well, can you go there?

LORI: Have you told him that, that he is the healthiest person in the system?

BRAD: (Shakes head yes)

LORI: That's nice.

TED: Be careful or he might use that.

BRAD: He already has.

TED: "Brad says I'm healthier than you, mom."

DEB: Yeah, that could bite ya'.

TED: Anything else for Brad, any thoughts? Brad, anything else?

BRAD: No, this was excellent, very good feedback.

DEB: Good luck.

BRAD: Especially the reframing—I appreciate that.

TED: Let us know. Lisa, do you want to share your case?

LISA: A 46-year old white female from a small town near Peoria, she is currently married, she has two children, she has a teenager that is from a previous relationship and a five-year-old from her marriage. The client originally came to me, which in and of itself is complicated, because she has a lot of physical problems. At one point, she was told by a doctor that she has RSD, which is a fatal muscular disease, if I understand that right, and she had deteriorated to the point where she and her husband actually planned her funeral and went and bought the casket, and then a doctor told her she didn't have RSD, and she started getting better, so she—there's a lot of somatic issues involved with everything, and that dates back to 1991. She started with carpal tunnel, and her symptoms got to the point where she was misdiagnosed with RSD, so there's a psychological piece there. Multiple, multiple chronic symptoms of PSD she talks about a lot. She—I did assessments for PSD—she had every symptom; I did assessments for major depression—she had every symptom; did assessment for hypermania—she had every symptom. She has trouble in every area of her life. My focus was in trying to help her see that all these physical symptoms either were—I am very careful—or largely emotional problems, and trying to get her to deal with the trauma. Severe physical abuse as a child from both parents, sexual abuse by a boyfriend at a point mom and dad were separated—you know, chronic abuse with boyfriends. Left home at a very early age, and was one of those kids living on the streets of Peoria, and would sleep with people to have a place to stay. The strongest connection that I have helped her to kind of reconnect to is one of the ways she survived is she would leave, as a child, would leave her house as early as she could get herself up and get things together, and go out into nature. She would be by a lake, she would be by trees. They became her family almost, the trees and the animals and the nature, and when we—I was trying to prepare her for Eye Movement Desensitization Reprocessing (EMDR), and her safe place was—which tells you how dissociative she can be—but the safe place—she used that skill, she was the eagle, she was looking through the eyes of the eagle and she could fly and see whatever she wanted to see, and the freedom and the power of that. So over time, I have tried to get her to reconnect with that skill, that ability, those resources, and she has, although she's disengaged from that as well. We start EMDR and we have some success and a lot of sabotaging behaviors, you know—just a few this year. She's created so much chaos, and she's done this with her son as well about "Will my insurance pay for therapy?" that she didn't have therapy for 5 months, and she's had insurance—she has Medicare—and they have paid for years for her to have therapy. She's on disability because of the mental health pieces. Another way that she disengages is currently—she approaches treatment and disengages is—she calls me for about 5 months—I wouldn't say regularly, but once a month, you know, "I want to come back, I know I need to start the EMDR, I know it helped, but I saw an ex-boyfriend, and I still had a panic response," and you know, I try to explain to her there is so much trauma, you know, working on one little piece is not going to make the trauma response go away. She's got herself—as a result of having that trauma reaction to seeing an ex-boyfriend—rarely leaving the house at this point, so she's taken the anxiety and added—almost, not completely—an agoraphobia piece to it, yet another obstacle for her to get better, and kind of a theme. It's not all the time, and sometimes I forget about it, and then she reminds me—part of staying sick; there's a payoff for her.

LORI: Absolutely.

LISA: She—there's a lot of payoffs, but one of them is maintaining this disability. Sometimes she'll call me, and for a while I'm confused—like, "Why do you want to document this?" She'll call me and, "I need you to document this symptom; this is a symptom I am having," and I'm like, "Okay," and then later it dawns on me that she'll use me to write a report for disability, and she described to me recently that that disability is the only way she can stay in her marriage and feel—because it's the only way she feels she contributes—so if the disability leaves, "I will not be able to cope staying married," and he, her husband, although he is only at home like 2 hours a day—he works two full-time jobs—so he's not the emotional support she craves everywhere but is the most stable person that's ever been in her life, ever. So part of the difficulty in seeing a lot of movement is the things she does to sabotage treatment, you know, the severity and the chronicity of that, and span of the trauma's, and some of the trauma's she re-creates, and there's a very—I hesitate to say bizarre—spiritual religious piece, because I think there can be truth there, but with most things she takes it so far you're always trying to find what's reality and what's not reality, and the spiritual piece is the same. She believes as an adolescent that negative energy was sent to her and it's almost like a psychic rape occurred in her bedroom, so she has a strong belief that those negative energies kind of haunt her. A most recent example, which validated her need to stay home, was this stranger pulled up in her driveway, and she went out to and was talking to him, and she said she was fine, and he said, "I used to live here. How long have you lived in this house?" and "Is so and so still around here?" and she said, "I was fine until I touched him, and there was such negative energy I had to run into the house," and then her reaction to that—she calls the police. "This person was here, I don't know who he was"—called all of her neighbors, so all of her neighbors—you know, she's calling again and distraught, totally traumatized because of this negative energy that she feels. My hesitation—you know, I am always trying to—you know, validate. Yes, people can have negative energy; yes, people can sense that, but that doesn't mean you're going to be attacked—you know, trying to balance, you know, her reality with the hypervigilance and the PTS stuff, and part of the struggle is, we may use an entire session just trying to talk about that, so we're not working on getting rid of the trauma, and often that happens. We use a session to talk about things that have happened, instead of working on resolving why they happen.

BRAD: She's a moving target.

LISA: Absolutely, and it can happen even in a benign conversation. You know someone can say something to her, and by the time she gets home, you know it could've been this very negative connotation, and she's traumatized by that conversation.

LORI: Lisa, has she had a psychiatric assessment; I mean is she on medication?

LISA: A couple, a couple. Well, that was many, many sessions; she was refusing to get on meds. I even brought her husband in, explaining to him why, you know, the physical aspects of what's happening to her and the need for medication. I don't know if it was to humor me or not, but she went to a psychiatrist; he did prescribe her an SSRI; of course, it made her feel totally awful, so she was on it like days. She—one positive thing is after that she found an agency—I don't know if that's the right word—a company—a business that tested her and could show her the chemical imbalances that I was talking to her about—the serotonin, the dopamine, the norepinephrine—and they gave her, you know, diet, and supplements to raise the serotonin, and she did start doing better. The only negative with that, she was doing better, so she stopped coming to treatment, but eventually she stopped all that and started getting sick again, and then, you know, started calling me again. So she refuses to take psychotropic meds, and I think many people have tried to get her to over the years. But she did have a psychological—this one—there's been several, because of her involvement in the different community stuff in 1995.

BRAD: Just those two issues?

LISA: A lot of borderline characteristics, histrionic characteristics. I wouldn't say she was one or the other, but you know just stuff all over the place that makes it difficult for her to have relationships with people. A lot of times, she gets angry because of something they said and that's horrible because—and then she's isolated.

BRAD: Multiple treatment experiences with other therapists?

LISA: Yes.

BRAD: Ever been in dialectical behavioral therapy?

LISA: Not that I know of. I know my experience is—she'll go, she'll seek—since I've known her, she's probably tried two different therapists—and then leaves them and comes back to me—that she kind of just goes from one person to the other.

LORI: You're the best so far, huh?

LISA: Well, I'm the current—let me say that—I'm the current one, and she doesn't feel like she can come into therapy because, you know, I would view her as grotesque because of where she is as far as her coping and what's going on with her now, but she'll talk to me on the phone. We've had two sessions on the phone.

TED: Does she have any awareness of the access to issues and how they impact her life, or have those been kept from her?

LISA: You know I think at one treatment time we were trying to get to there, but I don't think she has a lot of understanding, and when she gets education and gets some understanding, she loses that information somehow. I've tried to help her understand PTSD for a year and a half now, and she still says, "I don't understand, you need to help me understand."

LORI: Well, I mean this might be the same thing, but give her something like a Millon and you can graph out the results for her; at least she kind of has a pictorial of these are the things that might be affecting her life every second of the day . . .

LISA: Right.

LORI: . . . if they're strong personality disorders.

LISA: I think there is.

TED: I think that's probably the source of all the behavior you're talking about, the obstruction, but it feels like obstruction . . .

LISA: Right.

TED: . . . the therapy and changing that and persisting and all of that stuff. The trauma sure is there also, but if those other things are going to happen, they're going to happen, and you're just going to sabotage any attempts at sustaining—

LISA: Right.

TED: —the trauma. In fact the trauma may be very overwhelming, I am guessing—

LISA: Right.

TED: —for her to think about approaching, let alone dealing with daily life issues. The medication, her avoidance of medication, concerns me too, because you get worried about, you know, her ability to manage her mood, and—

LISA: Right.

TED: —and how is that going to help her be effective in applying anything she's learning?

LISA: The supplements and the diet did help.

TED: Yeah.

LISA: But she didn't sustain it, she didn't keep with it.

BRAD: Well, and because she's—no, she's not invested in getting well. She's got catch-22's kind of built in all around her, almost like a fortress.

LISA: Right. You know each avenue, medically, why that avenue is not a possibility to her because of all the medical symptoms. She kept—she's probably been to 50 doctors.

TED: RSD.

LISA: Yeah, and as a result of that, then trying to help her with medications, she developed some addiction issues, had to go to treatment, which totally traumatized her, and she had to leave, you know, she could not cope with it, so she's now—one of her fears is the fear of doctors. Although it did get her to a psychiatrist, but she doesn't trust what anyone says to her that is going on with her, except the visual of the serotonin deficits has stuck. She says, "I know I need the supplements to treat that."

TED: You said visual, so visual is important to her. She needs to see things.

LISA: Proof.

LORI: That's why I thought the Millon; you could plot out that, you could have it in front of her. That's the first thought I had, but the second one was—

LISA: That's a good idea because to try and talk about the sabotaging behavior, it always goes back to "You don't understand what it's like for me," you know.

BRAD: This is how she takes it: she fills out the questions and the reports in front of her, and it's interpreted to her, but it's her report.

TED: You need to take it really slow with her, and not the whole graph, but piece by piece.

BRAD: One session for one piece.

TED: I guess I find myself thinking about rapport, boy, rapport, rapport, rapport with her, just getting her to walk with you or you walk with her somehow, a lot of that is probably what she liked about the imagery and—

LISA: Every session I feel I am on a balance of trying to keep that rapport, but be direct enough to keep moving. Every session I feel that.

TED: Eighty percent or 90 percent rapport; maybe 10, maybe max 20 percent intervention. . . .

BRAD: And it's teaching intervention, not confrontation intervention.

LISA: Right.

BRAD: Just teaching.

LORI: I think you said something else, though, that she doesn't feel like she trusts very many people, but for some reason, Lisa, she trusts you because she keeps coming back to you.

LISA: Right.

LORI: Even—you know, she tries everyone else out, but she—"That Lisa, I'll keep going back to her, there's just something about her."

TED: So there's some basis there, that's good.

LORI: Yeah.

LISA: Well, I think it's a spiritual thing because we talked a lot about the eagle and nature, and the Native American spirituality, and I didn't think that was stupid, like her mother would've, or I agreed with her and we talked about that a lot. I think that's a piece.

JULIE: And I guess what stands out to me, what you were saying also was the negative energy and she believes that very strongly, and so maybe going with that, and also, you know, going with her, and saying, "Okay, yes—negative energy. What does she do to combat that with positive energy?" I mean other than just calling her neighbors and doing that—that's just giving in to the negative energy.

TED: Avoiding it and running away and—

JULIE: What is she doing? You know what is she doing for positive energy?

LISA: Right.

DEB: That the negative energy will overtake her.

LISA: And find her.

DEB: Is it the devil?

LISA: It came to her house.

DEB: Yeah, does she give it that frame? Is it evil? Is it the devil?

LISA: That's the—I think that's the association.

DEB: Okay.

LORI: See, I think I go back to Julie's comment about "Then let's find some positive energies that can protect you from the negative energies when they come."

LISA: Right.

JULIE: And that has nothing to do with her health—her, you know, social situation, or whatever.

LISA: That's what the nature piece was, when she was engaged the time before last, and she started going out to Wild Life Prairie Park and would work with the eagles and the owls, and there's a hawk out there, and she loved it. You know, she got herself a little leather glove and she would exercise them, and she did really well then, but now she can't go because she can't get out of the house.

LORI: How sad; they must miss her. I'd go there, "Boy, those animals must miss you."

LISA: Although that's not completely true. She—the guy that works with them asked her to go to a education presentation where he got to take the birds, and he asked her to go with him, and she did and had a blast, and that was pretty recent. She—so she's not in the house all the time. She'll go and help her husband when he's farming, you know, if he calls her and needs her. She'll go get her kids from school. I mean she's not always in the house, but the house will prevent her from getting better.

LORI: Uh-huh.

LISA: She can't go to treatment, and she can't go to—

TED: I wonder if she grows plants or raises animals—

LISA: I think she has animals.

TED: —or gets involved in nature things or Native American groups somehow or reading or something to build that resource for her.

LISA: Right.

LORI: Has she connected with or gone, like, to a tribal council or gone to a Native American drumming session? I mean, they have some of those out.

JULIE: Yeah.

BARBARA: Probably this weekend.

LORI: I mean, I think those might be really interesting.

LISA: I've tried to go there with her, and I'm not giving up on that by any means.

LORI: Sure.

LISA: But you know, I said earlier that the spiritual and religious pieces aren't really bizarre, but you think, "Oh, that's pretty—that's pretty weird". She's involved with the church, and even though she has these wonderful experiences with nature, she'll find where what we're saying as far as nature goes contradicts what her church says, and then that's—you know, that makes it evil.

LORI: Yeah.

LISA: You know, a couple of books on my bookshelf, she wouldn't ask me directly but tried to get me to get some books off of my bookshelf that her church would say are evil. You know, I just didn't do that, but she keeps coming back to that spiritual piece with me—so there's contradiction within her self—but won't say, won't make a decision.

DEB: Her instincts make it real.

LISA: Yeah.

JULIE: That parallels everything else she's doing—you know, the contradiction.

LISA: Yes, absolutely, absolutely.

TED: You can test for this, but I hear some schizotypal tendencies here, and a lot of looseness in her thinking.

LISA: A lot of looseness.

TED: And again, we're back to the role of medication at some point, with enough or more to help her maybe better manage that, but until then you can expect it to probably remain loose.

LISA: Right.

TED: I'm guessing.

DEB: But even with the PTSD, she's right in the middle of the retraumatization—

LISA: The hypervigilance—I mean, she'll lock all the doors and windows, and—

DEB: —and the physiology that goes with all that.

LISA: But the—so the main thing that I've heard is, you know, using the Millon to help with—

LORI: The picture piece.

LISA: —to help her understand what's happening to her, the visual, and to help get to a medication place possibly.

TED: Well, even more than that, I'd say it might even be too much for her right now, you know—rapport. Rapport.

LISA: Uh-huh.

TED: I mean, building this identity around her interests and her values and the nature stuff—I think that's the right direction to go for a long time, I think, and then maybe begin to edge—nonce you have that confidence to—you know, "Let's look at this picture a little bit more in a psychological side, or on—" But for now—boy, that would overwhelm her. I can see it overwhelming her. She'd run from it.

DEB: I think anything would.

BRAD: With the Axis II things going on, I think the most difficult thing with this is to keep the patient time frame of progress in your own head going through this, so you don't become impatient with your client going through this, because if you confront before you have rapport, that whole retraumatization piece gets filtered by her as rejection, or abandonment or criticism or mistrust, and it just starts the whole cycle over, so you have to be basically changing her time line to five times as long we can expect from any other client, before you actually get into that.

LISA: You know, when I was looking at her file this morning, I found a note. She'll often stop by, leave me a gift, leave me a note—she bought me flowers one time for my birthday—and I hadn't seen her in 6 months, but I found the note she had left, and then the note was about—you know, how appreciative she was and how helpful I was, but she's going to go see a counselor at Antioch—but if it doesn't go well, could she come back?

LORI: "I might come back to you. Well, just keep it, keep it just in case. I want you to like me, just in case, so I can come back."

LISA: Well, I'm wondering if it's that rejection piece, setting the dynamics up over and over—

LORI: Yeah.

LISA: —where I could tell her to not come back.

BARBARA: I'll test you.

BRAD: It's going to be a subtle place though, because she's giving you some clues here regarding the conflict between religiosity and your spirituality, and if she's going to Antioch group, it may be that it's not even you that's rejecting her—

LISA: Right, drawing in more confusion.

BRAD: —as it is much of what you represent.

LISA: Right.

JULIE: But I think you have an amazing opportunity because those books are just, you know, metaphors. She has—there might be something in your office that she doesn't agree with or that her church doesn't agree with, but then you have rapport with her, you're building a relationship, and so you're combating the way she looks at the world, that "there might be something negative, but I can still have a positive and growing relationship."

LISA: Make it all positive.

TED: We're at the end of our time folks. Any other thoughts for Lisa, closing thoughts?

DEB: It's very complicated.

TED: You know, I think rapport skills are really good with her, just keep working on those, I think. Well, I think that's our time for today. Thank you all for your participation, I hope you found something valuable, and let us know what happens, please.

LORI: Thank you, everybody.

LISA: Thank you, guys.

TED: Thanks.

Summary

Interest in group supervision among mental health practitioners has experienced a recent significant resurgence. Its potential to maximize resources, provide multidisciplinary feedback, and enhance overall staff development has fueled its application in many types of employment settings. Although the structural limitations and collegial dynamics of group supervision may not always lend themselves to in-depth individual case review, professionals can continue to supplement their supervisory needs through individual supervision. Effective group supervision requires skillful organizational and group facilitation skills, and the focus of issues to be addressed can range from case conceptualization and treatment planning to ethical dilemmas and the dynamics of the therapeutic relationship. Overall, group supervision provides a rich opportunity for clinical feedback, collegial support, professional education, and staff development.

Chapter Nine Final Discussion Questions

1. As a supervisor and supervisee, what would be your fears about being a member of group supervision? _____

   _____

   _____

   _____

2. What is your opinion about lifelong group supervision over your counseling career?

   _____

   _____

   _____

   _____

References

Bakes, A. J. (2005). The triadic working alliance: A comparison of dyadic and triadic supervision models. *Dissertation Abstracts International, 66,* 211A.

Borders, L. D. (1991). A systematic approach to peer group supervision. *Journal of Counseling & Development, 69,* 248–252.

Council for Accreditation of Counseling and Related Educational Programs. (2001). CACREP accreditation manual (2nd ed.). Alexandria, VA: Author.

Fall, M., & Sutton, J. M. (2004). *Clinical supervision: A handbook for practitioners.* Auckland, New Zealand: Pearson, Allyn & Bacon.

Granello, D. H., Kindsvatter, A., Granello, P. R., Underfer-Babalis, J., & Hartwig-Moorhead, H. (2008). Multiple perspectives in supervision: Using a peer consultation model to enhance supervisor development. *Counselor Education & Supervision, 9,* 32–48.

Hein, S., & Lawson, G. (2008). Triadic supervision and its impact on the role of the supervisor: A qualitative examination of supervisors' perspectives. *Counselor Education & Supervision, 48,* 16–31.

Linton, J. M. (2003). A preliminary qualitative investigation of group processes in group supervision: Perspectives of master's level practicum students. *The Journal of Specialist in Group Work, 28,* 215–226.

Nguyen, T. V. (2004). A comparison of individual supervision and triadic supervision. *Dissertation Abstracts International, 64,* 3204A.

Ray, D., & Altekruse, M. (2000). Effectiveness of group supervision versus combined group and individual supervision. *Counselor Education and Supervision, 40,* 19–30.

Russell-Chapin, L., & Ivey. A. (2004). *Your supervised practicum and internship: Field resources for turning theory into practice.* Pacific Grove, CA: Brooks/Cole.

Future Directions in Supervision

Improving Standards of Practice

Counseling licensure is now law in 50 states in America, Puerto Rico, and the District of Columbia (Neukrug, 2007; American Counseling Association, 2009). With it has come minimum educational standards and regulated supervision experience. Many states have begun to mandate continuing education to focus primarily on the critical issues surrounding counseling supervision. Although continuing education is a good thing, many of these efforts have fallen short. They are requiring a set amount of classroom hours and do not require continuation of direct counseling supervision.

It is the authors' opinion that required continuation of direct counseling supervision, post-licensure, is on the horizon. When it arrives, recommended continuing supervision will give way to mandated post-licensure supervision. This will strengthen our profession and improve standards of practice.

Discussion Question 1

Do you believe that mandatory supervision should be required of all licensed professionals? Explain. _____

_____

_____

_____

_____

_____

Spirituality

In a survey from The Polling Report (2004) responders acknowledge that 92 percent believe in God. Other national surveys reveal a high proportion of the population believes in something outside of themselves, a transcendent force (Aten & Hernandez, 2004). It makes sense, then, that counselors and supervisors will have clients with religious and spiritual concerns (Berkel, Constantine, & Olson, 2007). It also makes sense that supervisees and supervisors will have personal religious and spiritual concerns. Unfortunately, few graduate-level programs offer systematic training on religious or spiritual matters (Russell & Yarhouse, 2006; Conway, 2005; Brawer, Handal, Fabricatore,

OVERVIEW

The field of counseling supervision is in the midst of a golden renaissance due to many professional, economic, social, and technological factors. Counseling licensure has brought a renewed emphasis on maintaining good standards of practice. The high costs of health care and the influences of managed care have brought needed attention to counseling outcomes and efficient management of resources. The growth of counseling specialties and their expansion across many professional settings has generated a need for multidisciplinary approaches and applications. In addition, our society has made several significant cultural shifts. We are growing older and more diverse. Advances in technology have enriched our opportunities for speedy communication to remote areas via such modalities as e-mail, Internet2, teleconferencing, and group chat rooms. This final chapter discusses these numerous variables and new directions impacting the field of counseling supervision.

GOALS

- Explore new directions in clinical supervision
- Encourage helping professionals to engage in continued counseling supervision

Roberts, & Wajda-Johnston, 2002; Young, Cashwell, Wiggins-Frame, & Belair, 2002), and very little information occurs in the supervision literature on this matter (Bishop, Avila-Juarbe, & Thumme, 2003). However, according to Hicks (2009), helping supervisees in understanding their own personal beliefs, morals, and prejudices about different faiths is the first step in working effectively with others of different faiths. Much like in working with other areas of diversity, asking the client and/or supervisee up front is an essential feature in working with others of diverse faiths.

Discussion Question 2

Why do religion and spirituality seem to cause us such distress even in the realm of supervision?

_____

_____

_____

_____

_____

Live Supervision

Most counseling supervision is currently done well after the counselor and client have ended their sessions. This post mortem approach does allow the counselor and supervisor to review audio- and videotapes, reflect on what has transpired, and strategize new approaches for the next sessions; it does not allow for immediate feedback to the counselor, which could be used as immediate input on the counseling session.

In addition to the benefit of immediate feedback and therapeutic interventions, live supervision will often utilize doctoral and master's level students working conjointly with faculty in "supervision of supervision models." In one unique arrangement, predoctoral psychology interns working with master's-level social work interns were paired, allowing for greater flexibility, disruption of stubborn assumptions, and further personal growth opportunities (Haber, Marshall, Cowan, Vanlandingham, Gerson, et al., 2009).

Models of Training and Technology

Numerous models of supervision are offered in the previous chapters. Another model, family therapy supervision, however, has relied more exclusively on time, en vivo, and case supervision. One such model used by Steve DeShazer (1985) in their clinic is designed to teach the basic components of brief strategic therapy. Their training room is equipped with a two-way mirror or a direct line telephone across to the therapy room. Typically, one or more supervisors with other students in training observe live therapy behind the two-way mirror. At certain key moments, a call may come in from the observation room with suggested counseling interventions, which the counselor can immediately deliver to the client. The session can be debriefed immediately after its conclusion. This style has led to other more advanced technologies.

Receiving immediate feedback through technology has many advantages over the traditional supervision-type model. First, the critical moment is not lost. Second, many eyes, ears, and minds are focused on the therapy material, allowing for great depth and creativity to be harnessed for the client's benefit. Third, feedback to the counselor is immediate and its impact instantly observable. Most counseling offices and training centers are not designed to allow for two-way observation and direct communication from supervisee to supervisor. The future may hold expansion of the technology because it is so profound. Layne and Hohenshil (2005) assert that technology in counseling and supervision is here to stay. If this supervision method is here for the long run, then counseling training programs must provide the necessary workshops and courses to assist supervisees and supervisors (Vaccaro & Lambie, 2007). New interactive CDs are being developed to assist supervisees and supervisors in building skills (Baltimore, Fitch, & Gillam, 2005; Dufrene & Tanner, 2008; Manzanares, O'Halloran, McCartney, Filer, Varheley, et al., 2004). Studies indicate that already e-mail, computer-based teleconferencing, electronic mailing lists, chat rooms, computer-assisted live supervision, Internet2, videoconferencing for international practicums, and supervision are being implemented in many counseling and social work training programs (Harvey & Carlson, 2003; Panos, 2005; Ganor & Constantine, 2002). Damianakis, Climans, and Maziali (2008) used data from a 4-year study of web-based video conferencing with caregivers groups and weekly supervision. Even though there were some technological difficulties, results of the Internet group were consistent with those in face-to-face group settings.

These advances in technology have touched the counseling profession and have profound implications for facilitating new and exciting opportunities for counseling supervision. Not only can individuals communicate immediately online with e-mail and the Internet, but groups can also interact in real time to allow for true synchronous learning. Distance, time, and cost are all harnessed to serve the needs of the client, supervisee, and supervisors (Watson, 2003, 2005; Mallen, Vogel, & Rochlen, 2005). However, as technology increases, all helping professions must be aware of the "technologically inspired generation gap between new and established workers." (Csiernik, Furze, Dromgole, & Rishchynski, 2006, p. 9). There will have to be a concerted effort to bridge that gap.

Other technological advances include direct video streaming that allows the user to download one set of files, thus allowing clients in rural settings to access mental health services via computer video conferencing. Computer technology is not without its problems. The equipment is expensive; coordination between sites can be timely and is sometimes disrupted; and people are often reluctant to trust the technology or lack the technical skills to use it. The issues of confidentiality become even more complicated when using technology. The use of encrypted or secure transmission of supervisory information is essential (Shaw & Shaw, 2006).

The future of counseling supervision will no doubt capitalize on the benefits of these technologies for both individual and group supervision. They are efficient and useful tools for written, spoken, and visual communications (Kennedy, 2008).

Discussion Question 3

Share your beliefs about the advances in technology and their efficacy in counseling and supervision. _____

_____

_____

_____

_____

Multidisciplinary Supervision

No longer do counselors work only in small groups with other therapists. They work in schools with teachers and administrators, in health care settings with physicians and nurses, in churches with ministers and lay church employees, and even in agencies of multidisciplinary professionals. It is not uncommon for an agency or group practice to consist of counselors, social workers, psychologists, psychiatrists, and even paraprofessional volunteers. This diversity of perspectives is deeply enriching, but there are more opportunities for philosophical differences, turf battles, and professional arrogance. Davys and Beddo (2008) conducted a small qualitative investigation on interprofessional supervision and discovered that rather than hindering the learning process, the diversity of disciplines seemed "to enhance the breadth of learning and participants were challenged to clarify ideas and language" (p. 68).

Despite our differences, the future will likely bring an influx of multidisciplinary supervision, and this will be a positive development in the helping fields. Although great skill will be needed to successfully facilitate multidisciplinary supervision, the benefits far outweigh the potential disadvantages. Multidisciplinary supervision can build cohesiveness. It can allow an individual therapist the opportunity to alternative perspectives. It can also reduce the costs associated with more traditional one-on-one, face-to-face supervision.

Discussion Question 4

What are the potential supervisory benefits in having a multidisciplinary approach? _____

_____

_____

_____

_____

_____

Group Supervision

As the barriers of post-licensure counseling supervision diminish, more and more professionals will seek ongoing counseling supervision. Although many will likely continue to prefer a one-on-one supervision relationship, more will seek group supervision opportunities. Group supervision has many advantages over individual supervision (Ray & Altekruse, 2000). It pools the experiences and resources of several professionals and allows all to learn from vicarious and direct participation in the supervision process.

Group supervision may not be for everyone. It requires a certain level of personal confidence, security, and vulnerability to be effective. To bare your soul in front of your colleagues is no small task, but the benefits are great. For further information on group supervision, go back to Chapter Nine.

Group supervision can provide an expanded professional support network. It can save both time and money, as many professionals can benefit from the same supervision session and share the costs. In today's world of ever-increasing direct hours and increasing standards of practice, group supervision is sure to have a greater appeal to many professionals.

The social work profession has a wonderful history of conducting business in small groups. The idea of "partnered practice," in which the transfer of knowledge is among and between groups in therapy and supervision, may become an essential part of future supervision (Aronoff & Bailey, 2005).

Multicultural Focus

As the texture of our society changes, so too does the skill base needed to successfully counsel the increasingly diverse clients who seek our services. Today's clients are as diverse as the tapestry of America and the world. They are multicultural: African American, Asian, Caucasian, Latino, Hispanic, Indian, Middle Eastern. They are sexually diverse: heterosexual, bisexual, and homosexual. They are rich and poor, educated and uneducated, male and female, and young and old.

Counseling supervision must be aware of these diverse needs, communication styles, and differing beliefs and values. Our basic counseling theories and practices are not enough. A recent social constructionist model of supervision suggests that there should be two distinct goals in assisting supervisees and supervisors in becoming culturally relevant. The first goal is to better understand our differences rather than striving to be culturally competent. The second task is to encourage "insiders" (p. 70) to create their own directives in supervision (Hair & O'Donoghue, 2009).

Our future requires that we become citizens of the world, expand our knowledge of diverse populations, and know our limits as they affect the standards of care that we provide. Supervision will assist us in that endeavor.

Discussion Question 5

Generalize what we know about multicultural counseling to the world of supervision. What are some of the most important factors? _____

_____

_____

_____

_____

Geriatric Populations

We are getting older. By the year 2010, it is estimated that there will be 40 million people who are considered elderly. Census data indicates that individuals 65 and older are the fastest growing segment of the American population (Allied Health, 2003). Therefore, there is an increased demand for all helping professionals, including counselors, social workers, psychologists, and other health care professionals (Rizzo & Rowe, 2006). Not only are we older, but we are generally more literate than any previous generation. This has drastic implications for the counseling profession. The needs of the geriatric population have been well documented. They include transitions from work to retirement, more activity to less, ample to fixed incomes, and family focus to marital refocus, as well as eventual change and loss, health and decline, and everyday life "adjustments." Everything changes as we age, and the nature of our youth-focused culture is not easily sustained as we age. This is the challenge we all face.

Certification programs are springing up to specifically address the issues faced by this aging population. Counseling supervisors and their supervisees would be well advised to seek out those programs and arm themselves with the tools they need to help address these trends. The research overwhelmingly indicates that healthy aging is the rule, not the exception. It is imperative that helping professionals prepare ourselves to meet the needs of this aging population.

Discussion Question 6

Are the helping professions doing enough to prepare current and new counselors to deal with the aging population? How does this impact supervision? _____

_____

_____

_____

_____

Evidence-Based Treatment

Almost 20 years ago, when managed care extended its reach to mental health services, one of its primary goals was to promote the outcomes of mental health treatment. Outcomes were measured by both reduced costs and successfully achieved therapy goals. At the time, this sent shock waves through a profession that cherished the privacy of the counseling relationship and subjective nature of therapeutic outcomes.

Today, in many respects things have come full circle. We have learned from our managed care colleagues how to pay closer attention to therapeutic outcomes and counseling outcome research (Elliott, 2002). We now establish specific treatment goals, we provide a full multiaxial DSM-IV-TR diagnosis, and some of us use standardized measures of therapeutic outcomes, from simple pre–post therapy checklists to more sophisticated computerized software programs.

Although many managed care companies have let up on their more rigid functions such as external treatment plan documentation, reauthorization providers, and limited treatment authorizations, the counseling profession is refocusing on evidence-based treatment, or "What works for whom and when?" A future trend in counseling supervision will be refinement of therapeutic techniques and procedures and their applications for specific clients with specific problems. The need to know that what we are doing is effective will go far in improving our standards of care.

Stoltenberg and Pace (2007, 2008) discuss the need for competency-based supervision approaches that can be viewed as extensions of the counseling skills models that flourished in the late 1960s and 1970s. The need for defining what competency-based skills look like and what defines competency-based supervision is clearly where the supervision field is headed (Falendar & Shafranske, 2004, 2007). The microcounseling supervision model (MSM) illustrated in Chapter 7 of this book is an excellent example of competency-based supervision (Russell-Chapin, 2007). Another essential dimension of competency-based supervision is to ask supervisees "to investigate and use approaches or interventions that have some empirically established rationale or, lacking that, strong theoretical grounding, and then assess how and why this approach works or doesn't work for them when implemented with a given client" (Stoltenberg & Pace, 2007).

Discussion Question 7

How will competency-based supervision change current supervision practices? _____

_____

_____

_____

_____

_____

Brain Research

In the last decade, there have been many advances in brain research and understanding how and why the brain functions. This research debunks some old ideas, validates other existing beliefs, and offers new and encouraging interventions for helping people grow and learn. All of this information has many new implications for the field of counseling and counseling supervision.

For years, educators and helping professionals believed that the brain matured around 12 years of age. Now with the help of functional magnetic resonance imaging (fMRI), researchers know that the adolescent brain is fully developed by around 25 years of age. However, neuroscientists now understand that the brain has the capability to adapt and develop new living neurons up until the very end of our lives, according to Dr. Norman Doidge (2007), a psychiatrist at Columbia University Center for Psychoanalytic Training and Research in New York. This process is called neuroplasticity. "Neuroplasticity can result in the wholesale remodeling of neural networks.... a brain can rewire itself, state authors Schwartz and Begley in their 2003 book called *The Mind and the Brain: Neuroplasticity and the Power of Mental Force.*

The brain is no longer considered a stagnant organ, but 3 pounds of plastic, fluid, and malleable tissue. Human beings can change their brains and develop new pathways through repetition and learning new skills. Challenging and taxing the brain with new tasks such as learning a foreign language can forge different pathways in the brain. The capacity to restructure our brain allows our brain span to match our life span. The old adage "you can't teach an old dog new tricks" no longer holds true. This information is so important to the field of counseling and supervision because the counseling world finally has empirical evidence showing why cognitive counseling works. Through MRIs, we can finally see pre- and post-test evidence that shows the impact of counseling on the brain. With negative plasticity, the neuronal pathways often lead to faulty thoughts and behaviors. With new thoughts and practice, clients are taught to build new neuronal pathways or positive plasticity, and change the brain toward healthier functioning (Schwartz & Begley, 2003). This holds true for clients, counselors, supervisees, and supervisors.

With this emerging brain research comes numerous new questions. How will this information be utilized? Will neuroscience research impact our effectiveness and efficiency? Supervisors and child and youth workers in a social skills program created a therapeutic program answering just those questions and demonstrating brain research's utility.

The authors combined recent neurobiology, developmental psychology, and evidenced-based strategies to help high-risk children (Fraser & Robinson, 2009).

Discussion Question 8

What beliefs about counseling and supervision are challenged by the newest advances in brain research? _____

_____

_____

_____

_____

Increasing Demand

Other strong directions in our profession are the increasing demand for counseling services, the pressure to hold insurance reimbursement rates low, working with Medicare and Medicaid, and the increasingly difficult time counselors are having maintaining their previous levels of income (Rizzo & Rowe, 2006). We are a profession under unprecedented attack from both our own success and the continual escalation of U.S. health care costs. Although mental health services account for only less than 1 percent of the total U.S. health care budget, our reimbursement rates have been held unchanged for the last 10 years. This creates a nearly impossible dilemma for mental health providers.

As previously noted, we have done a terrific job in lessening the demand for services and the corresponding drain on the U.S. health care budget. Something has to give, and looking into the future suggests it will be the counseling professional.

Many counselors chose their professions as a vocational calling. They wanted to help others, but increasing demands and soaring costs force some to find another line of work. Some augment their clinical caseload with fee-for-service consultation work. Some seek administrative positions. Some teach. Others are closing their careers altogether. Increased demand is a future crisis for professional counselors. Counseling supervision throughout the life span of our counseling careers could support us through this crisis (Russell-Chapin, 2007).

Discussion Question 9

What are your concerns about increasing demands for counseling and supervision and the high costs associated? _____

_____

_____

_____

_____

Professionalization of Supervision

The final future direction in counseling supervision is the continuing professionalization through professional organizations, the establishment of standards of practice, specialized training programs, and required continuing education in supervision for licensed professionals. Soon gone will be the day that supervision is optional or that any well-intended professional can call him- or herself a counseling supervisor.

Another method gaining popularity, because of necessity, wisdom, and effectiveness, is the use of mandatory supervision policies, supervision plans, and professional wills. These documents clarify all expectations of supervision for the supervisees and supervisors, offer directions for supervision, and ensure that clients' and colleagues' needs are met if something unexpected happens to the helping professional. The examples of a supervision policy and plan provided in Chapter One and the professional will shown below are just that—examples. These are the documents the authors use in their private practice. Each practitioner owes it to him- or herself, clients, family members, and other members in the agency or private practice to responsibly handle the expectations of supervision and of a sudden death or disability (Ragusea, 2002). The Clinical Supervision Policy spells out specifically what is expected in supervision from the supervisor, supervisee, and other team members. The Supervisory Plan offers unique direction for the specific needs of the supervisee. The professional will is a provision that gives authority and explicit instructions to a professional executor of all essential information regarding the private practice or agency client files. Usually, the executor is a mental health colleague who knows the counselor and agency well. Holloway (2003) outlines a few additional topics for inclusion: current and past client records, billing and financial information, appointment book location, e-mail addresses and needed passwords, keys location for files, patient notification, liability insurance policy numbers, and how to notify the carrier.

PROFESSIONAL WILL OR EXECUTOR INSTRUCTIONS
FOR THE DISPOSITION OF CLIENTS OF _____, IN THE
EVENT OF DEATH, DISAPPEARANCE OR DISABILITY

A. The Professional Executor

_____ and/or
The Staff of Resource Management Services, Inc.
3020 W. Willow Knolls
Peoria IL 61614
(309) 681-5652

B. My Attorney

_____
_____
_____
_____

C. My Accountant

_____
_____
_____
_____

(Continued)

D. General Information

- Office location: _____
- Keys to my office and file cabinets are located: _____
  _____ _____
- Closed client files are located: _____
- Open client files are kept: _____
- My personal appointment book is kept: _____
  _____ _____
- Billing records are kept by the Professional Executor.
- License, malpractice policy, and managed care contracts are kept by the Professional Executor.
- All client records must be handled only by the Professional Executor.
- The Professional Executor will assist in notification and/or therapeutic issues to be addressed with my clients.
- Billing issues, insurance, and other administrative details already handled by the Professional Executor will continue to be handled by them.

E. Specific Instructions to the Professional Executor

1. In the event I am unable to work for more than 2 weeks but can communicate effectively, please contact me about how to proceed. Whatever we discuss at that time will take precedence over this document.

2. In the event of my death, disappearance, or in the event of temporary or permanent decisional incapacitation, the Professional Executor should take the following steps:

   a. Telephone all scheduled clients and notify them of my current circumstances. Assess clients' need for ongoing therapy. After review of my treatment notes and your telephone assessment, make professional referrals as appropriate. If the client accepts the referral please obtain the client's consent to release the records to the designated therapist. Please attend to insurance or managed care needs requirements.

   b. When clinically appropriate, please offer my clients one face-to-face contact to process my death or incapacitation with them. If they cannot afford it or the insurance company denies such a session, cover the costs from my outstanding earned salary or bill my estate.

3. Copies of referred clients' records should be forwarded to their new therapists. All remaining records should be maintained and/or destroyed as is customary by the Professional Executor and as advised by the guidelines of the American Psychological Association.

4. Please defer to my designee, _____, or executor of my estate, _____, any financial decisions to be made regarding outstanding bills or compensation that is due. If a review of the clinical file is needed to ascertain the outstanding earnings due, please conduct such a review and inform my estate executor of the resulting amounts.

5. Please notify in writing all managed care or insurance companies of my circumstances.

6. There are three copies of this Professional Executor Instructions. The first is located with my other personal papers _____. The second is held by the Professional Executor. The third is on file with my attorney.

7. Charge my estate for the cost of professional time and other reasonable expenses incurred as the result of these instructions.

8. This professional living will is established and shall be governed by the laws of the state of Illinois. I intend that this power of attorney be universally recognized and admissible in any jurisdiction.

_____	_____
Therapist	Date
_____	_____
Professional Executor	Date
_____	_____
Witness	Date

Discussion Questions 10

1. How will policies such as a supervision will and supervision plans assist in professionalizing the field of supervision? _____

_____

_____

_____

2. In your opinion, are these policies even necessary? _____

_____

_____

_____

Summary

Professional, economic, social, and technological factors have impacted the development of counseling supervision. Most of the future directions speak to a promising new era; however, a few challenges remain. The momentum is building to ride the wave of reduced stigmas, unprecedented access, and the professionalization of supervision. The challenges are real. How do we establish a code of conduct among all mental health workers that values the role of continuing post-licensure supervision? How do we ride the economic pressures that have increased our workload and frozen salaries? How do we effectively equip ourselves with the knowledge and skills to service a diverse and changing population? And how do we take advantage of the incredible opportunities of technological advances while remaining a human-oriented profession? The answer to these questions will shape our future and the future of counseling supervision.

The Association for Counselor Education and Supervision of the American Counseling Association, Division 16 of the American Psychological Association, and the National Association of Social Workers are all working hard to elevate and promote the status and role of the clinical supervisor in their respective professional associations. The future for counseling supervision is bright. It is likely that the next 5 to 10 years will see a substantial increase in the number of full-time professional counseling supervisors. We are witnessing the birth of a new related profession. The challenge is up to each of us to accept and seek the best type of supervision (Baird, 2002).

Chapter Ten Final Discussion Questions

1. What additional supervisory directions do you foresee? _____

_____

_____

_____

_____

2. Which of the discussed directions meet your supervision needs? _____

_____

_____

_____

_____

References

American Counseling Association. Retrieved October 2009 from www.counseling.org.

Allied Health. (2003). 32, 18–26.

Aronoff, N., & Bailey, D. (2005). Partnered practice: Building on our small group tradition. *Social Work with Groups, 28,* 23–39.

Aten, J. D., & Hernandez, B. C. (2004). Addressing religion in clinical supervision: A model. *Psychotherapy: Theory, Research, Practice, Training, 41,* 152–160.

Baird, B. N. (2002). *The internship, practicum, and field placement handbook.* (3rd ed.). Upper Saddle River, NJ: Prentice Hall.

Baltimore, M. L., Fitch, T., & Gillam, L. (2005). Interactive CD-ROM development for use in research: A study of clinical supervision. *Journal of Technology in Counseling, 4.* Retrieved January 2009 from http://jtc.colstate.edu/Vol4_1/Index.htm

Berkel, L. A., Constantine, M. D., & Olson, E. (2007). Supervisor multicultural competence: Addressing religious and spiritual issues with counseling students in supervision, *The Clinical Supervisor, 26,* 3–15.

Bishop, D. R., Avila-Juarbe, E., & Thumme, B. (2003). Recognizing spirituality as an important faction in counselor supervision. *Counseling and Values, 48,* 34–46.

Brawer, P. A., Handal, P. J., Fabricatore, A. N., Roberts, R., & Wajda-Johnston, V. A. (2002). Training and education in religion/spirituality with APA-accredited clinical psychology programs. *Professional Psychology: Research & Practice, 33,* 203–206.

Conway, E. M. (2005). Collaborative responses to the demands of emerging human needs: The role of faith and spirituality in education for social work. *Journal of Religion and Spirituality in Social Work, 24,* 65–77.

Csiernik, R., Furze, P., Dromgole, L., & Rishchynski, G. (2006). Information technology and social work-the dark side or light side? *Journal of Evidence-Based Social Work, 3,* 9–26.

Damianakis, T., Climans, R., & Marziali, E. (2008). Social workers' experiences of virtual psychotherapeutic caregivers groups for Alzheimer's, Parkinson's, Stroke, Frontotemporal dementia and traumatic brain injury. *Social Work with Groups, 31,* 99–116.

Davys, A. M., & Beddoe, L. (2008). Interprofessional learning for supervision: "Taking the blinkers off." *Learning in Health & Social Care, 8,* 58–69.

DeShazer, S. (1985). *Keys to solution in brief therapy.* New York: W. W. Norton.

Doidge, N. (2007). *The brain that changes itself.* New York: Penguin Books.

Dufrene, R. L., & Tanner, Z. (2008). Multimedia CD: Play therapy counseling skills. *Journal of Technology and Counseling, 5.* Retrieved January 2009 from http://jtc.colstate.edu/Vol5_1/Dufrene.htm

Elliott, R. (2002). Hermeneutic single-case efficacy design. *Psychotherapy Research, 12,* 1–21.

Falender, C. A., & Shafranske, E. P. (2004). *Clinical supervision: A competency-based approach*. Washington, DC: American Psychological Association.

Falender, C. A., & Shafranske, E. P. (2007). Competence in competency-based supervision practice: Construct and application. *Professional Psychology: Research and Practice, 383*, 232–240.

Fraser, M., & Robinson, B. (2009). Bridging child and youth work with brain research: Enhancing social and academic learning opportunities for developmentally-at-risk children. *Relational Child & Youth Care Practice, 22*, 64–72.

Ganor, K. A., & Constantine, M. G. (2002). Multicultural group supervision: A comparison of in-person vs. Web-based formats. *Professional School Counseling, 6*, 104–121.

Haber, R., Marshal, D., Cowan, K., Vanlandingham, A., Gerson, M., & Fitch, J. (2009). "Live" supervision of supervision: "Perpendicular" interventions in parallel processes. *Clinical Supervisor, 28*, 72–90.

Hair, H. J., & O'Donoghue, K. (2009). Culturally relevant, socially just social work supervision: Becoming visible through a social constructivist lens. *Journal of Ethnic & Cultural Diversity in Social Work, 18*, 70–88.

Harvey, V. S., & Carlson, J. F. (2003). Ethical and professional issues with computer-related technology. *School Psychology Review, 32*, 92–104.

Hicks, M. (2009). Religious/spiritual matters not to be ignored. *The National Psychologist, 18*, 17.

Holloway, J. D. (2003). Professional will: A responsible thing to do. *APA Online Monitor, 34*. Retrieved January 2009 from www.apa.org/monitor/feb03/will.aspx

Kennedy, A. (2008). Plugged in, turned on and wired up. *Counseling Today, 8*, 34–38.

Layne, C. M., & Hohenshil, T. H. (2005). High tech counseling: Revisited. *Journal of Counseling and development, 83*, 222–226.

Mallen, J. J., Vogel, D. L., & Rochlen, A. B. (2005). The practical aspects of on-line counseling: Ethics, training, technology and competency. *The Counseling Psychologist, 33*, 776–818.

Manzanares, M. G., O'Halloran, T. M., McCartney, T. J., Filer, R. D., Varhely, S. C., & Calhoun, K. A. (2004). CD-rom technology for education and support of site supervisors. *Counselor Education and Supervision, 43*, 220–231.

Neukrug, E. (2007). *The world of the counselor*. (3rd ed). Pacific Grove: CA, Brooks/Cole.

Panos, P. T. (2005). A model for using videoconferencing technology to support international social work field practicum students. *International Social Work, 48*, 834–841.

Polling Report, The. (2004). FOX News/Opinion Dynamics Poll, September 23–24, 2003. Retrieved January 2009 from www.pollingreport.com/religion.htm

Ragusea, S. A. (2002). A professional living will for psychologists. In L. VandeCreek & T. L. Jackson (Eds.), *Innovations in clinical practice: A source book* (pp. 301–305). Sarasota, FL: Sarasota Professional Resource Press.

Ray, D., & Altekruse, M. (2000). Effectiveness of group supervision versus combined group and individual supervision. *Counselor Education and Supervision, 40*, 19–30.

Rizzo, V. M., & Rowe, J. M. (2006). Studies of the cost-effectiveness of social work services in aging: A review of the literature. *Research on Social Work Practice, 16*, 67–73.

Russell, S. R., & Yarhouse, M. A. (2006). Religion/spirituality within APA accredited psychology predoctoral internships. *Professional Psychology: Research and Practice, 37*, 430–436.

Russell-Chapin, L. A. (2007). Supervision: An essential for professional counselor development. In J. Gregoire & C. M. Jungers (Eds.), *The counselor's companion: What every beginning counselor needs to know* (pp. 79–80). Mahwah, NJ: Lawrence Erlbaum.

Schwartz, J., and Begley, S. (2003). *The mind and the brain: Neuroplasticity and the power of mental force*. NY: HarperCollins.

Shaw, H. E., & Shaw, S. F. (2006). Critical ethical issues in online counseling: Assessing current practices with an ethical intent checklist. *Journal of Counseling & Development, 85*, 41–53.

Stoltenberg, C. D., & Pace, T. M. (2007). The scientist-practitioner model: Now more than ever. *Journal of Contemporary Psychotherapy, 37*, 195–203.

Stoltenberg, C. D., & Pace, T. M. (2008). Science and practice in supervision: An evidence-based practice in psychology approach. In W. B. Walsh (Ed.) Biennial Review 06 Counseling Psychology, Vol. 1. Oxford, England: Taylor & Francis.

Vaccaro, N., & Lambie, G. W. (2007). Computer-based counselor-in-training supervision: Ethical and practical implications for counselor educators and supervisors, *Counselor Education & Supervision, 47*, 46–56.

Watson, J. C. (2003). Computer-based supervision: implementing computer technology into the delivery of counseling supervision. *Journal of Technology in Counseling, 3*. http://jtc.colstate.edu/vol3_1/Watson/Watson.htm

Watson, J. C. (2005). Factors influencing the online learning efficacy beliefs of counselors in training. *Journal of Technology in Counseling, 4*. Retrieved January 2009 from http://jtc.colstate.edu/Vol14_1/indes.htm

Young, J. S., Cashwell, C., Wiggins-Frame, M., & Belair, C. (2002). Spiritual and religious competencies: A national survey from CACREP-accredited programs. *Counseling and Values, 47*, 22–23.

Information Packet Forms

PRACTICUM/INTERNSHIP CONTRACT

This agreement is made on _____ by and between
month/day/year

_____ and the Human Development Counseling
Field Site

Program at _____. The agreement is effective for a period
Institution

from _____to _____ for a minimum of
month/day/year   month/day/year

750 clock hours. Hours worked during University holidays and breaks will be determined by the student and site based on the needs of school or agency.

The Human Development Counseling Program agrees:

1. to assign a University faculty liaison to facilitate communication between the University and the site.

2. to provide a profile of the student, an academic calendar, and a course syllabus for Practicum/Internship.

3. to notify the students that they must adhere to the administrative policies, rules, standards, schedules, and practices of the site.

4. that the faculty liaison shall be available for consultation with both site supervisors and students.

5. that the University supervisor is responsible for the assignment of a course grade.

6. that the student carries liability insurance in the amount of $1,000,000/$3,000,000 during the entire time this agreement is in effect.

The Practicum/Internship site agrees:

1. to assign a practicum supervisor who has the appropriate credentials, time, and interest for training the student.

2. to provide opportunities for the student to engage in a variety of counseling activities under supervision and for evaluating the student's performance.

3. to provide the student with adequate work space, telephone, office supplies, and staff to conduct professional activities.

4. to provide supervisory contact, which involves some examination of student work using audio/videotapes, observation, and/or observation.

5. to provide written evaluation of student's work based on criteria established by the University Program.

_____

____

Name   Address   Phone   SS#

will be the primary site supervisor. The training activities checked below will be provided in sufficient amounts to allow an adequate evaluation of the student's level of competence in each activity.

_____ will be

Name   Phone

the faculty liaison with whom the student and practicum site supervisor will communicate regarding progress, problems, and performance evaluation.

PRACTICUM/INTERNSHIP ACTIVITIES

___ Individual Counseling
personal/social/educational/
occupational

___ Career Counseling

___ Group Counseling
co-leading
leading

___ Supervision
individual
group
peer

___ Intake Interviewing

___ Case Conferences
staff meetings

___ Testing
administration
analysis/interpretation

___ Psychoeducational Activities
parent conferences
outreach programs

___ Consultation

_____   _____

Site Supervisor   Date

(INSTITUTION) PROGRAM OF STUDY

WEEKLY TIME SCHEDULE   *WEEK #*

* = Direct Service Hours

Date	Location	Amount of Time*	Practicum/Internship Activity	Comments
____	_____	_____	_____	_____
____	_____	_____	_____	_____
____	_____	_____	_____	_____
____	_____	_____	_____	_____
____	_____	_____	_____	_____
____	_____	_____	_____	_____
____	_____	_____	_____	_____
____	_____	_____	_____	_____
____	_____	_____	_____	_____
____	_____	_____	_____	_____
____	_____	_____	_____	_____
____	_____	_____	_____	_____
____	_____	_____	_____	_____

TOTALS:

This Week: **Semester:**

Total Hours: _____   Total Hours: _____

Direct Service Total: _____   Direct Service Total: _____

CLIENT INFORMED CONSENT FORM

I,_____,
agree to be counseled by a practicum/intern student in the (Program) at
(Institution). I further understand that I may participate in counseling interviews
that will be audiotaped, videotaped, and/or viewed by practicum/intern students
through the use of one-way observation windows. I understand that I will be
counseled by a graduate student who has completed advanced course work in
counseling. I understand that the student will be supervised by a faculty member
of the (Institution) (Program) and an agency site supervisor.

Client's Signature: _____

Date of Birth: _____ Today's Date: _____

Counselor's Signature: _____

Effective Date: _____

Expiration Date: _____

CLIENT RELEASE FORM

I agree for my child, _____, to be counseled during the (date) school year by _____, Counselor Intern in the (Program) at (Institution). I understand that my child may participate in counseling interviews that may be audiotaped or videotaped, and/or viewed by practicum/internship students through the use of one-way observation windows. I further understand that _____ has completed advanced coursework in counseling/therapy and will counsel my child. I further understand that a (Institution) Professor and an on site (Institution) supervisor will oversee the Counselor Intern.

_____ I agree for my child to be counseled by the Counselor Intern for the (date) school year and for those sessions to be videotaped or audiotaped.

_____ I agree for my child to be counseled by the Counselor Intern for the (date) school year; however, I do not wish for those sessions to be videotaped or audiotaped.

_____ I agree to have counseling information shared with: _____

                                                        Person(s)

Parent/Guardian Signature _____ Date _____

Student Signature _____

Counselor Intern Signature _____ Date _____

Date Effective _____ Date Contract Expires _____

Site Supervisor's Evaluation of Student Counselor's Performance

Suggested Use: This form is to be used to evaluate overall performance in counseling. The form will be completed twice per term by the onsite supervisor. The form is appropriate or individual or group counseling.

Name of Student Counselor: _____

Name of Supervisor/Agency: _____

Date of Evaluation: _____

Period Covered by the Evaluation: _____

DIRECTIONS: The supervisor is to circle the number that best evaluates student counselor performance in each category.

General Supervision Comments

	Requires Assistance	Acceptable Performance	Exceptional Performance
1. Demonstrates a personal commitment in developing professional competencies..	12	34	56
2. Invests time and energy in becoming a counselor..............................	12	34	56
3. Accepts and uses constructive criticism to enhance self-development and counseling skills................................	12	34	56
4. Engages in open, comfortable, and clear communication with peers and supervisors..	12	34	56
5. Recognizes own competencies and skills and shares these with peers and supervisors..	12	34	56
6. Recognizes own deficiencies and actively works to overcome them with peers and supervisors................................	12	34	56
7. Completes case reports and records punctually and conscientiously..	12	34	56

The Counseling Process

	Requires Assistance	Acceptable Performance	Exceptional Performance
8. Researches the referral prior to the first interview............................	12	34	56
9. Keeps appointments on time..	12	34	56
10. Begins the interview smoothly..	12	34	56
11. Explains the nature and objectives of counseling when appropriate..	12	34	56
12. Is relaxed and comfortable in-the interview....................................	12	34	56
13. Communicates interest in and acceptance of the client..................	12	34	56
14. Facilitates client expression of concerns and feelings......................	12	34	56

General Supervision Comments

	Requires Assistance	Acceptable Performance	Exceptional Performance
15. Focuses on the content of the client's problem................................	12	34	56
16. Recognizes and resists manipulation by the client...........................	12	34	56
17. Recognizes and addresses positive affect of the client....................	12	34	56
18. Recognizes and addresses negative affect of the client....................	12	34	56
19. Is spontaneous in the interview..	12	34	56
20. Uses silence effectively in the interview..	12	34	56
21. Is aware of own feelings in the counseling session...........................	12	34	56
22. Communicates own feelings to the client when appropriate.........	12	34	56
23. Recognizes and skillfully interprets the client's covert messages......	12	34	56
24. Facilitates realistic goal-setting with the client...............................	12	34	56
25. Encourages appropriate action-step planning with the client...	12	34	56
26. Employs judgment in the timing and use of different techniques..	12	34	56
27. Initiates periodic evaluation of goals, action-steps, and process during counseling...	12	34	56
28 Explains, administers, and interprets tests correctly.......................	12	34	56
29. Terminates the interview smoothly..	12	34	56

The Conceptualization Process

	Requires Assistance	Acceptable Performance	Exceptional Performance
30. Focuses on specific behaviors and their consequences, implications, and contingencies...	12	34	56
31. Recognizes and pursues discrepancies and meaning of inconsistent information..	12	34	56

	Requires Assistance	Acceptable Performance	Exceptional Performance
32. Uses relevant case data in planning *both* immediate and long-range goals...	12	34	56
33. Uses relevant case data in considering various strategies and their implications...	12	34	56
34. Bases decisions on a theoretically sound and consistent rationale of human behavior..	12	34	56
35. Is perceptive in evaluating the effects of own counseling techniques...	12	34	56
36. Demonstrates ethical behavior in the counseling activity and case management..	12	34	56

Additional comments/suggestions to improve performance:

_____

_____

_____

_____

_____

_____

_____

Date:_____ Signature of Supervisor: _____

My signature indicates that I have read the above report and have discussed the content with my site supervisor. It does not necessarily indicate that I agree with the report in part or in whole.

Date:_____ Signature of Student Counselor: _____

Web Addresses for Professional Organizations and Codes of Ethics

American Association of Christian Counselors: Code of Ethics
http://www.aacc.net/code.html

American Association of Marriage and Family Therapy: Code of Ethics
http://www.aamft.org/about

American Association of Pastoral Counselors: Code of Ethics
http://www.aapc.org/content/ethics

American Counseling Association: Code of Ethics and Standards of Practice:
http://www.counseling.org/Resources/Codeofethics/TP/Home/CT2.aspx

American Group Psychotherapy Association: Guidelines for Ethics
http://www.groupsinc.org/group/ethicalguide.html

American Medical Association: Principles of Ethics
http://www.ama-assn.org

American Psychoanalytic Association: Principles and Standards of Ethics for Psychoanalysts
http://www.gpsa.org/ethics90l.html

American Psychological Association: Ethical Principles and Code of Conduct
http://www.apa.org/ethics/code/index.aspx

Australian Psychological Society: Code of Ethics
http://www.psychology.org.au/about/ethics/

American School Counseling Association: Principles for Professional Ethics
http://www.schoolcounselor.org

British Association for Counselling: Code of Ethics and Practice for Counsellors
http://www.bacp.co.uk/ethical_framework/

Canadian Counselling Association: Codes of Ethics
http://www.ccacc.ca/coe.html

Canadian Psychological Association
http://www.cpa.ca

Commission on Rehabilitation Counselor Certification: Code of Professional Ethics
http://www.crccertification.com/pages/crc_ccrc_code_of_ethics/10.php

Ethics Updates
http://ethics.sandiego.edu

National Association of Alcoholism and Drug Abuse Counselors: Ethical Standards
http://www.naadac.org/index.php?option=com_content&view=article&id=185&Itemid=113

National Organization for Human Service Education: Ethical Standards
http://www.nohse.com/ethstand.html

National Association of Social Workers: Code of Ethics
http://www.naswdc.org/pubs/code/default

National Board for Certified Counselors: Code of Ethics
http://www.nbcc.org/ethics/NBCCethics.htm

New Zealand Association of Counsellors Inc.: Code of Ethics
http://www.nzac.org.nz/ethics.html

Counseling Interview Rating Form

Counselor:_____ Date:_____

Observer:_____ Tape #:_____

Observer:_____ Audio or Video (please circle)

Supervisor:_____ Session #:_____

For each of the following specific criteria demonstrated, make a frequency marking every time the skill is demonstrated. Then assign points for consistent skill mastery, using the ratings scales below. List any observations, comments, strengths, and weaknesses in the space provided. Providing actual counselor phrases is helpful when offering feedback.

Ivey Mastery Ratings

3 Teach the skill to clients (teaching mastery only)

2 Use the skill with specific impact on client (active mastery)

1 Use and/or identify the counseling skill (basic mastery)

Each skill marked by an X should be seen consistently on every tape.

To receive an A on a tape, at least 52–58 points must be earned.

To receive a B on a tape, at least 46–51 points must be earned.

To receive a C on a tape, at least 41–45 points must be earned.

Specific	Frequency	Comments	Skill Mastery Rating
A. Opening/Developing Rapport			
X **1.** Greeting			
2. Role Definition/Expectation			
3. Administrative Tasks			
X **4.** Beginning			
B. Exploring Phase/Defining the Problem Micro Skills			
1. Empathy/Rapport			
2. Respect			
X **3.** Nonverbal Matching			
X **4.** Minimal Encourager			
X **5.** Paraphrasing			
X **6.** Pacing/Leading			
X **7.** Verbal Tracking			
X **8.** Reflect Feeling			
X **9.** Reflect Meaning			
10. Clarifications			
11. Open-Ended Questions			
X **12.** Summarization			
X **13.** Behavioral Description			
X **14.** Appropriate Closed Question			
X **15.** Perception Check			
X **16.** Silence			
X **17.** Focusing			
X **18.** Feedback			
C. Problem Solving/Defining Skills			
X **1.** Definition of Goals			
X **2.** Exploration/Understanding of Concerns			
X **3.** Development/Evaluation of Alternatives			
4. Implement Alternative			
5. Special Techniques			
6. Process Counseling			
D. Action Phase/Confronting Incongruities			
1. Immediacy			
2. Self-Disclosure			
3. Confrontation			
4. Directives			
5. Logical Consequences			
6. Interpretation			
E. Closing/Generalization			
1. Summarization of Content/Feeling			
2. Review of Plan			
3. Rescheduling			
4. Termination of Session			
5. Evaluation of Session			
X **6.** Follow-up			
F. Professionalism			
1. Developmental Level Match			
2. Ethics			
3. Professional (punctual, attire, etc.)			

G. Strengths:

H. Areas for improvement:

Glossary of Counseling Interview Rating Form Skills

Opening/Developing Rapport Skills

Definition	Intention
Greeting: A simple acknowledgment to the client	Build rapport
Role Definition/Expectation: Description of the counselor roles and intention of counseling; confidentiality and its limit	Provide structure
Administrative Tasks: Procedures necessary for counseling such as client rights; payment; scheduling and intake forms	Clarify procedures
Beginning: An open-ended question demonstrating to the client the interview is starting, such as "What do you want to work on today?"	Offer an expansive method of beginning the interview

Exploration Phase/Defining the Problem/Microskills

Definition	Intention
Empathy/Rapport: Behaviors and attitudes indicating understanding and active listening	Encourage the client to continue
Respect: Offering genuine acknowledgment of client's concerns	Build rapport
Nonverbal Matching: Using body gestures and positions to mirror the client's	Build rapport and acceptance
Minimal Encourager: An occasional word or "uh-huh" encouraging the client to continue	Encourage the client to continue
Paraphrasing: Actively rephrasing in the counselor's own words and perceptions what the client has stated, such as "Your mother died recently and you miss her."	Create understanding of client's words
Pacing/Leading: Allowing the client to direct the interview flow by counselor matching of words and verbal intonation; counselor directing when interview flow needs transition	Encourages comfort, discourages resistance
Verbal Tracking: Consistent following of client's verbal direction and themes	Create continuity from client's content
Reflect Feeling: Paraphrase the client's feelings, such as "How sad that must be."	Increases understanding of client's feelings
Reflect Meaning: Paraphrasing the client's deeper level of experience, such as "Death can be an ending and perhaps a beginning."	Increases wider perspective
Clarifications: Eliminating confusion of terms by seeking clearer understanding of client's words	Eliminates confusion of terms
Open-Ended Questions: Asking global questions for the purpose of receiving maximum or infinite amount of information, such as "What do you miss the most about your mother?"	Receives maximum or infinite amount of information
Summarization: Paraphrasing a cluster of themes or topics during the interview, providing transition and/or closure	Provides for transition and/or closure
Behavioral Description: Informing the client of what you observe of a behavior or mannerism; "When we began talking about sister and mother's relationship, I noticed your eyes teared up and you moved your chair away from me.	Eliminates assumptions about behaviors and assists in client awareness
Appropriate Closed Questions: An intentional question used to obtain a finite amount of information, such as "How old were you when your mother died?"	Gains finite amounts of information

Continued

Continued

Perception Check: A periodic moment to ask the client whether your perceptions or ideas about the concern are accurate; "Is that accurate concerning your sister and mother's relationship?"	Check counselor's perception and accuracy
Silence: Allowing purposeful, quiet reflection during the interview	Allows for purposeful, quiet reflection during the interview
Focusing: Consistent and intentional selection of topic, construct, and/or direction in the session	Aids in direction of the session
Feedback: Offering information to the client concerning attitude and behavior, such as "Last week you came here with crumpled clothes, but today you have washed your hair and clothes."	Provides awareness about behaviors, thoughts, and feelings

Problem-Solving Skills/Defining Skill

Definition	Intention
Definition of Goals: Statements stipulating directions, outcomes, and goals of the client	Stipulates directions for counseling
Exploration/Understanding of Concerns: Using needed microskills to discover the nature of the concern	Collects essential information about client's concern
Development/Evaluation of Alternatives: Assisting the client in creating a myriad of options for problem solution; assessing the potential and possibilities surrounding each option	Assesses the potential and possibilities surrounding each option
Implement Alternative: Actively planning and articulating necessary steps for placing option into reality	Assists in putting ideas into action
Special Techniques: Any counseling intervention used to assist the client in deeper understanding of the concern, such as imagery or an Empty Chair	Provides for the needs of individual clients
Process Counseling: Helping the client understand special themes and dynamics involved in the problem, such as loss and fear	Allows for deeper understanding of client issues

Action Phase/Confronting Incongruities

Definition	Intention
Immediacy: Stopping the interview and immediately seeking clarification about a dynamic or observation in the client or between the counselor and client; "You stopped talking after your Dad was mentioned. What is happening right now?"	Keeps the sessions in the here and now
Self-Disclosure: Offering relevant, helpful, and appropriate information about the counselor for the purpose of client assistance; "When my father died, I was 21 years old. My compass was gone, and I was lost."	Assists the client in universality of life
Confrontation: Pointing out client discrepancies between words, behaviors, thoughts	Helps the client to become aware of thoughts and actions
Directives: An influencing statement specifying an action or thought for the client to take; "The next time you visit your mother's grave, I suggest you write a poem expressing your fears and loneliness."	Offers needed structure for differing developmental client needs; shows acceptance
Logical Consequences: Explaining the results/consequences of the client's actions and solutions; the consequences can be natural or logical.	Points out results of client's decisions
Interpretation: Presenting a new frame of reference on the client's concern possibly through different theoretical orientations; "It may be that the death of your mother forces you to be alone with yourself and your own fears."	Presents a new frame of reference on the client's concern

Closing/Generalization

Definition	Intention
Summarization of Content/Feeling: Closing the session by tying together themes involving subject matter and emotions	Ties together the counseling themes
Review of Plan: Organizing the desired outcome into a plan and reviewing it with the client	Reminds the client of previously discussed ideas
Rescheduling: Arranging for another session if needed	Provides additional counseling opportunities
Termination of Session: Offering appropriate generalizations from counseling to the client's outside world when goals have been achieved	Brings counseling outcomes to the real world
Evaluation of Session: Asking the client to reflect on the essentials of each interview; "What will you take from today's session that will assist you between now and our next meeting?"	Provides tangible counseling outcomes for the client and counselor
Professionalism: Making appropriate professional decisions following unwritten and written organizational mores and guidelines	Adds respect to counselor and client

Professionalism

Definition	Intention
Developmental Level Match: Assessing the client's developmental level and selecting counseling interventions accordingly	Creates intentional responses corresponding to client needs
Ethics: Following a set of ethical guidelines provided by a professional organization; making appropriate ethical decisions	Assists in remaining prudent in decision-making process

Practice Supervision Scenarios

Instructions: Read through the five case presentations. Each is formatted using a case presentation standardized guide. Analyze the supervisory question with the case information. Select the "best fit" model for each situation. At the end of each case, there are several discussion questions to assist in your decision making. The authors' preferred choices are also presented at the end of the book.

Case Presentation Guide 1

I. Introduction

   a. Abbreviated Name of Client: Jenny

   b. Age: 27

   c. Gender: Female

   d. Presenting Problem(s) in Client's Words: Jenny is mad at her father because he wants her to move out on her own. Jenny is also sad that her main friends all have boyfriends and don't have as much time for her anymore.

      Present Signs and Symptoms: The client has had three angry outbursts at her retail job and in the last 3 months has not left her room during the weekends.

   e. Multicultural Domain Issues: Caucasian

II. History

   a. Present Problem(s)

      1. Onset: The problem began when Jenny entered graduate school.

      2. Duration: She has been in school for 1 full year.

III. Past History of Psychiatric Illness

   There is no past psychiatric history.

IV. Contributing Medical Illness

   Jenny is dealing with a form of muscular dystrophy.

V. Brief Family History

   Jenny is the older of two children. She has a younger brother who is 25 years of age. Her mother and father have been married for 30 years.

VI. Social History

   a. Martial Status: Jenny is single and does not have a boyfriend.

   b. Employment: Jenny is a full-time graduate student and is working a retail job.

   c. Current Living Arrangements: Jenny is living back at home until she graduates from her program of study.

VII. DSM-IV-TR Diagnosis on Five Axes

    a. Axis I: Presenting Problems and Focus of Clinical Attention—309.28

    b. Axis II: Personality Disorders/Mental Retardation—v71.09

    c. Axis III: Relevant Medical Concerns—359.1

    d. Axis IV: Psychosocial Stressors—v62.89

    e. Axis V: Global Affective Functioning (GAF)—85

VIII. Wellness Focus

    a. Physical: Jenny is exercising at least two times per week for 30 minutes.

    b. Spiritual: She is Protestant and attends church once per week.

    c. Occupational: Jenny is a student.

    d. Social: Jenny has friends and goes out at least once a week.

    e. Emotional: Her emotional needs are being met through family and friends.

    f. Intellectual: Jenny is studying and obtaining a master's degree.

IX. Prognosis

    a. Poor

    b. Fair

    c. Good: Jenny's prognosis is "Good," as she is in personal counseling and has been receptive to the counseling process and new skills.

X. Treatment Goals in Specific and Measureable Terms

    a. To learn the concepts of assertiveness training

    b. To respectively assert her thoughts and feelings to one family member and friend each week

XI. Supervisee's Supervision Needs and Wants/Supervision Question

I honestly was paralyzed when the client expressed her frustrations about her father. I asked a question immediately that didn't even seem relevant. My Supervision Question: What should I do when I get lost in counseling and don't even know what skill to use?

1. Based on this case presentation and the supervisory question, which of the five supervision models may be the best fit?

_____

_____

_____

_____

2. Explain your selection process.

_____

_____

_____

_____

3. How might this model assist you in working with this supervisee?

_____

_____

_____

_____

Authors' Preferred Model

Based on the supervisory question and case presentation, the microcounseling supervision model would be an excellent way to conduct this supervision session. Using the CIRF would assist the supervisee in better understanding the micro- and macrocounseling skills and even process her fears about being lost in the counseling session.

Review from Chapter Seven

Basic Tenet

- Supervisees benefit from a standardized, atheoretical approach assisting them in reviewing, offering feedback, and evaluating micro- and macrocounseling skills and the counseling interview.

When to Use

- When essential microskills are not effectively utilized, selecting the microcounseling supervision model is suggested.

Supervisor's Roles and Behaviors

- Use the Counselor Interview Rating Form (CIRF) as a mechanism for creating a reciprocal supervision process for offering constructive feedback.
- Choose from the three MSM components based upon supervisee's needs: Reviewing Skills with Intention, Classifying Skills with Mastery, and Processing Supervisory Needs.

Supervisor's Emphasis and Goals

- Assist the supervisee with clarifying and defining all micro- and macrocounseling skills.
- Identify and classify observed skills with intention using the CIRF.
- Process the strengths and liabilities of the counseling session answering the supervisory question.

Supervisee's Growth Areas

- The supervisee begins to better understand and classify all microcounseling and macrocounseling skills.
- The supervisee progresses to the mastery level of skill development.

Limitations

■ The major limitation is that MSM is best utilized when there is a videotape or digital tape of a counseling session. In some settings obtaining a recording of a counseling session does not easily occur.

Case Presentation Guide 2

I. Introduction

   a. Abbreviated name of Client: Karl

   b. Age: 42

   c. Gender: Male

   d. Presenting Problem(s) in Client's Words: My wife committed suicide, and I found her.

   e. Present Signs and Symptoms: Karl is overwhelmed with his parenting responsibilites. He has difficulty sleeping and cries often during the day.

   f. Multicultural Domain Issues: Caucasian

II. History

   a. Present Problem(s): His wife of 20 years committed suicide after the third suicide attempt. He is now a single parent of three children, ages 17 (male), 13 (female), and 10 (male).

      1. Onset: His bereavement has continued, with severe depressive symptoms.

      2. Duration: There has been a 1-year anniversary of his wife's death.

III. Past History of Psychiatric Illness

   There was one episode of counseling when Karl was shot down during the Iraq war.

IV. Contributing Medical Illness

   There are no contributing medical illnesses.

V. Brief Family History

   Karl and his family have traveled during their marriage of 20 years. Karl was in the military. He and his wife, Meredith, had three children. Meredith had a history of depression and two other suicide attempts. When Karl was injured in the Iraq War, he left the military to settle down.

VI. Social History

   a. Martial Status: Karl is a widower.

   b. Employment: Karl is currently working as a civilian as an engineer.

   c. Current Living Arrangements: Karl and his children live in the family home.

VII. DSM-IV-TR Diagnosis on Five Axes

   a. Axis I: Presenting Problems and Focus of Clinical Attention—v62.82; 309.81

   b. Axis II: Personality Disorders/Mental Retardation—v71.09

   c. Axis III: Relevant Medical Concerns—NA

   d. Axis IV: Psychosocial Stressors—v61.20

   e. Axis V: Global Affective Functioning (GAF)—60

VIII. Wellness Focus

   a. Physical: Karl exercised on a daily basis. The family struggles with eating together and eating a balanced diet.

   b. Spiritual: The family practices Catholicism and attends church regularly.

   c. Occupational: Karl is not satisfied with his engineering job.

   d. Social: Karl is willing to help others but has very few friends.

   e. Emotional: Karl has difficulty expressing his emotions.

   f. Intellectual: He is bright and dedicated but is not challenged in his current job.

IX. Prognosis

   a. Poor

   b. Fair

   c. Good: The prognosis for Karl is "Good," if he continues to work through his grief and corresponding depression.

X. Treatment Goals in Specific and Measureable Terms

   a. Talk to his children about their mom's life in the next month.

   b. Understand the two types of grieving: instrumental and intuitive.

   c. Examine the root of his depression.

   d. Establish weekly family discussions and a family routine.

XI. Supervisee's Supervision Needs and Wants/Supervision Question

   During the second session with my client, he shared some very personal concerns and became vulnerable during the session. My immediate response was to be direct and offer advice. I was uncomfortable. My Supervision Question: What do I need to do differently so I don't panic? How can I become more comfortable with feelings?

1. Based on your knowledge of the supervision models and the supervision questions, which model may be the best fit for this supervision session?

_____

_____

_____

2. Please explain your selection process.

_____

_____

_____

3. What components of the selected model will assist you the most in helping this supervisee? Be specific.

_____

_____

_____

Authors' Preferred Model

Based on the Supervision Question and the case presentation, interpersonal process recall (IPR) would be an excellent preferred choice for this supervision session. This model allows for safe yet gentle questions to explore and lead the supervisee's feelings, thoughts, and experiences about the counseling interaction. The skill of immediacy allows the supervisee to examine "what's occurring now during the counseling session."

Review from Chapter Eight

Basic Tenet

- Supervisees need an environment where they can safely analyze their communication styles and strategies.

When to Use

- If a supervisee seems to be stuck in the counseling interview, this method allows for safe, immediate feedback and a chance to reflect on the counseling experience.

Supervisor's Roles and Behaviors

- Stop the videotape at any time to discuss essential personal and/or counseling issues. If a videotape is not available, lead the supervision session with needed questions.

Supervisor's Emphasis and Goals

- The main goal is to stop a counseling videotape or supervisory session and use the skill of immediacy to gently discover counseling blocks, styles, and experiences.

Supervisee's Growth Area

- The supervisee has immediate feedback to assist in safely understanding the strengths and liabilities of the counseling interview.

Limitations

- This supervision approach is best used with video or digital recordings, so the supervisor can start and stop the interview when processing is required. However, a variation of IPR can be used without recordings, by asking the supervisee to recall how he or she felt at that moment.

Case Presentation Guide 3

I. Introduction

    a. Abbreviated name of Client: Gwen

    b. Age: 68

  c. Gender: Female

  d. Presenting Problem(s) in Client's Words: I was diagnosed bipolar many years ago. I am not taking any medications now. Last week I was in a meeting and there was a difficult crisis discussed. I could feel myself getting agitated. My regular coping strategies didn't seem to work.

  e. Present Signs and Symptoms: Gwen is exhibiting signs of anxiousness and irritation.

  f. Multicultural Domain Issues: Caucasian

II. History

  a. Present Problem(s): Gwen was diagnosed with Bi-Polar Disorder I.

  b. Onset: Twenty years ago, after their fourth child, Gwen had several manic episodes.

  c. Duration: Through proper medication early on and learned skills, Gwen has been living a well-balanced life.

III. Past History of Psychiatric Illness

  Until the first manic episode and one divorce in 1976, Gwen had not had any history of psychiatric illness.

IV. Contributing Medical Illness

  Gwen had a recent physical last week. She is in excellent health.

V. Brief Family History

  Gwen has had four children and two husbands. Her father was an alcoholic. She has been married for 20 years to her second husband.

VI. Social History

  a. Martial Status: Married

  b. Employment: Gwen is recently retired from a business/financial career.

  c. Current Living Arrangements: She and her husband, Gary, live together.

VII. DSM-IV-TR Diagnosis on Five Axes

  a. Axis I: Presenting Problems and Focus of Clinical Attention—309.00; 296.4

  b. Axis II: Personality Disorders/Mental Retardation—301.81

  c. Axis III: Relevant Medical Concerns—250.00

  d. Axis IV: Psychosocial Stressors—v61.10

  e. Axis V: Global Affective Functioning (GAF)—75

VIII. Wellness Focus

  a. Physical: Gwen exercises every morning.

  b. Spiritual: Her spiritual life is important to her, and she practices a protestant (Methodist) religion on a regular basis.

  c. Occupational: Gwen enjoys volunteering.

  d. Social: She and Gary are active in a country club and flower club.

  e. Emotional: Gwen is able to communicate her thoughts and feelings on a consistent basis.

  f. Intellectual: Gwen is an avid reader.

IX. Prognosis

    a. Poor

    b. Fair

    c. Good: Gwen's prognosis is "Good." She knew to come back to counseling when this event triggered her agitation.

X. Treatment Goals in Specific and Measureable Terms

    a. Explore what details of this meeting triggered Gwen.

    b. Identify what coping skills Gwen has continued to use and what skill she needs to use to maintain her healthy state of balance.

XI. Supervisee's Supervision Needs and Wants/Supervision Questions

I believe my conceptualization of this client's treatment has gone well. My main intervention seemed to go well. My Supervision Questions: Am I on the right track, and what else should I be looking for to be even more effective with this client?

1. Based on your knowledge of the supervision models and the supervision questions, which model may be the best fit for this supervision session?

_____

_____

_____

_____

2. Please explain your selection process.

_____

_____

_____

_____

3. What components of the selected model will assist you the most in helping this supervisee? Be specific.

_____

_____

_____

_____

Authors' Preferred Model

Based on the supervision question and the case presentation, any developmental model would serve the supervisee well. Using the Stoltenberg, McNeil, and Delworth developmental supervision model, the first supervisory task would be an assessment of the supervisee's developmental level. In this case, the supervision questions direct the supervisor to level 2.

This shows the supervisee moving toward independence yet needing encouragement from the supervisor. The growth areas needing attention may be interventions, skill competency, and client conceptualization.

Review from Chapter Four

Basic Tenet

- According to the Stoltenberg, McNeil, and Delworth's developmental supervision model, supervisees grow at individual paces, with differing needs and styles of learning, often with stages of growth that are dependent upon skill level and need of the client.

When to Use

- Use this model when assessment of the developmental level of the supervisee is needed and surmised.

Supervisor's Emphasis and Goals

- Assess the supervisee's developmental level of functioning from levels 1 through 4
- Understand the supervisee's world, motivational levels, and degree of autonomy
- Identify needed growth areas in each of the four levels, using the nine intervention areas listed below

Supervisor's Roles and Behaviors

Level 1	Beginning	Supervisor models needed skills and behaviors and plays the role of teacher.
Level 2	Intermediate	Supervisor provides some structure but also encourages exploration.
Level 3	Advanced	The supervisor listens and offers suggestions when asked.
Level 4	Master Counselor	The supervisor provides collegial and consultation functions.

Supervisee Growth Areas

1. Interventions
2. Skill competence
3. Assessment techniques
4. Interpersonal assessment
5. Client conceptualization
6. Individual differences
7. Theoretical orientation
8. Treatment goals and plans
9. Professional ethics

Limitations

■ This model does not go deep enough into specific supervision methods for each supervisee level, and it focuses only on student development as supervisees (Haynes, Corey, & Moulton, 2003).

Case Presentation Guide 4

I. Introduction

  a. Abbreviated name of Client: Rod

  b. Age: 20

  c. Gender: Male

  d. Presenting Problem(s) in Client's Words: I went on a church mission and was away from home for the first time. I was having difficulty making decisions and sleeping.

  e. Present Signs and Symptoms: Rod is displaying signs of anxiousness and has lost 10 pounds.

  f. Multicultural Domain Issues: Hispanic

II. History

  a. Present Problem(s): Rod was home schooled through high school. One outside resource suggested he may have Attention Deficit Disorder. It was never assessed. All males in the family have taken a church mission out of high school. Rod went to Central America, and mission officials said Rod was having difficulty following through with directives and tasks.

    1. Onset: Mom noticed sleeping concerns at around 5 years of age.

    2. Duration: Presently Rod is averaging 4 hours of sleep per night and eating three meals a day but losing weight.

III. Past History of Psychiatric Illness

  Rod has never had any psychiatric illness.

IV. Contributing Medical Illness

  Rod has no contributing medical illness.

V. Brief Family History

  Rod is the only child. Mom was a teacher but quit her job to home school. Mom is very involved in Rod's life. Dad is employed at a large production plant that makes tractors.

VI. Social History

  a. Martial Status: Single

  b. Employment: Not employed

  c. Current Living Arrangements: Rod is living at home right now.

VII. DSM-IV-TR Diagnosis on Five Axes

  a. Axis I: Presenting Problems and Focus of Clinical Attention—314.9; 300.02

  b. Axis II: Personality Disorders/Mental Retardation—301.6

  c. Axis III: Relevant Medical Concerns—NA

  d. Axis IV: Psychosocial Stressors—v61.20; v62.3

  e. Axis V: Global Affective Functioning (GAF)—50

VIII. Wellness Focus

    a. Physical: Rod is active in sports, especially basketball.

    b. Spiritual: The family is very involved in the Mormon Church.

    c. Occupational: He is not working but did have a paper route with Mom.

    d. Social: He enjoyed the friends on his basketball team. Rod stated his mission partner was very nice, and he misses him.

    e. Emotional: Rod wants to do what is right and complete his mission. He doesn't want to talk about his having to come back home.

    f. Intellectual: Rod passed all his home school equivalency tests. He doesn't enjoy school, but he does want to go to a local community college after his mission is completed.

IX. Prognosis

    a. Poor

    b. Fair: Rod's prognosis is "Fair." Becoming self-sufficient will be a slow process, and with proper family support Rod can learn those skills.

    c. Good

X. Treatment Goals in Specific and Measureable Terms

    a. A genogram history will be taken and developed in the first interview session.

    b. Rod will be assessed for ADD/ADHD in the next 2 weeks.

    c. Rod will see a psychiatrist for possible medications in the next 2 weeks.

    4. Learning a new emotional regulation skill will be presented each week.

XI. Supervisee's Supervision Needs and Wants/Supervision Questions

I often use a genogram to obtain needed information. This time it seems like I am missing a connection. My Supervision Questions: What piece of the puzzle might I be missing? How can I expand the effectiveness of genograms?

1. Based on your knowledge of the supervision models and the supervision questions, which model may be the best fit for this supervision session?

_____

_____

_____

2. Please explain your selection process.

_____

_____

_____

3. What components of the selected model will assist you the most in helping this supervisee? Be specific.

_____

_____

_____

Authors' Preferred Model

Based on the supervision questions and the case presentation, a theoretical specific model of supervision may be the best fit. In this case, a family systems Bowenian supervision model would be demonstrated within the supervisory session.

Review from Chapter Five

Basic Tenet

- The basic tenet of Bowen's generational family systems supervision model stresses the importance of the emotional system of the family unit.

When to Use

- Use this approach when the supervisee needs to better understand his client, not in isolation, but within the entire family system.

Supervisor's Roles and Behavior

- The supervisor may work on the main constructs of the supervision sessions, using correlating counseling techniques such as genograms, triangulation, and differentiation.
- The supervisor acts as a teacher and coach.

Supervisor's Emphasis and Goals

- The main goal is to understand how the client reacts and responds within an entire family system.

Supervisee Growth Areas

- The supervisee will learn personal and client areas of family dysfunction and possible relationships needing healing.

Limitations

- This supervision model may address the client's and supervisee's family system, but it may not address the personal needs of the client.

Case Presentation Guide 5

I. Introduction
   a. Abbreviated name of Client: Susan
   b. Age: 38
   c. Gender: Female
   d. Presenting Problem(s) in Client's Words: My boss suggested I enter into counseling because of work concerns.

    e. Present Signs and Symptoms: Susan appears anxious in the office. She doesn't look the counselor in the eyes. She states she doesn't sleep well and eats poorly. Her circle of friends is limited to two.

    f. Multicultural Domain Issues: Caucasian

II. History

    a. Present Problem(s): Susan's boss says she is cranky and doesn't get along well with others.

        1. Onset: Susan says her problems this time began about 6 months ago.

        2. Duration: Susan says she may be depressed every day for the past 6 months.

III. Past History of Psychiatric Illness

She has never been hospitalized and never been to a previous counselor.

IV. Contributing Medical Illness

Susan was diagnosed with breast cancer last year. Her cancer is now in remission.

V. Brief Family History

Her parents are still married unhappily. Susan has an older sister and brother. Susan is living alone with a dog and cat.

VI. Social History

    a. Martial Status: Susan is single and never had a boyfriend.

    b. Employment: Susan has a high-paying occupation as a lawyer.

    c. Current Living Arrangements: Susan lives alone.

VII. DSM-IV-TR Diagnosis on Five Axes

    a. Axis I: Presenting Problems and Focus of Clinical Attention-296.32

    b. Axis II: Personality Disorders/Mental Retardation—301.83

    c. Axis III: Relevant Medical Concerns—NA

    d. Axis IV: Psychosocial Stressors—v62.2

    e. Axis V: Global Affective Functioning (GAF)—60

VIII. Wellness Focus

    a. Physical: There is very little exercise or activity.

    b. Spiritual: She was reared Catholic but is not practicing.

    c. Occupational: Her job is stressful and challenging.

    d. Social: She has two friends, but Susan reported being on the "outs" with both of them.

    e. Emotional: Susan doesn't express her thoughts and feelings directly. She does report sending anonymous gifts and messages to people.

    f. Intellectual: Susan is bright and a dedicated worker.

IX. Prognosis

    a. Poor

    b. Fair

    Susan's prognosis is "Fair," if she will consistently attend counseling. Structured sessions and times are needed. However, once Susan commits to biweekly sessions, a crisis occurs and she quits counseling. She has quit four times thus far in one year.

    c. Good

X. Treatment Goals in Specific and Measureable Terms

    a. Understand and articulate the criteria for Borderline Personality

    b. Practice during our sessions the material presented from Dialectical Behavior Therapy

    c. Commit to directly expressing her emotions at least one time each counseling session

    d. Go over the results of the MCMI-III

XI. Supervisee's Supervision Needs and Wants/Supervision Questions

Somehow I have allowed this client to gradually creep into my personal life too much. My Supervision Questions: How did I let this occur? And I want to explore what strategies I have already implemented and what other boundaries might be necessary.

1. Based on your knowledge of the supervision models and the supervision questions, which model may be the best fit for this supervision session?

_____

_____

_____

2. Please explain your selection process.

_____

_____

_____

3. What components of the selected model will assist you the most in helping this supervisee? Be specific.

_____

_____

_____

Authors' Preferred Model

Based on the supervision questions and the case presentation, the social roles supervision models provide an effective strategy. Using the discrimination supervision model would assist the supervisee in answering her oncerns and questions. In this case, the supervisee is requesting assistance focusing on the process and conceptualization of the counseling session. The supervisor's role would be that of teacher and counselor.

Basic Tenet

■ Supervisees benefit from those supervisors who work from multiple theoretical orientations and focus on supervisee's needs by being able to respond flexibly with any needed strategy, technique, and/or guidance based upon the supervisor's role and focus.

When to Use

- When the supervisee is unaware of own experience with clients, the discrimination model assists in expanding counseling knowledge base.

Supervisor's Roles and Behaviors

- The supervisor responds flexibly with needed role of teacher, counselor, and/or consultant.
- The supervisor selects the necessary focus.

Supervisor's Emphasis and Goals

- Emphasize two primary functions during each supervision session, that of the supervisor's role and focus.
- Three supervisor roles selected based upon supervisee needs are teacher, counselor, and consultant.
- Each of these roles has three areas of focus for skill-building purposes.
- The three areas of focus are process, conceptualization, and personalization.

Limitations

- There is limited empirical evidence testing the efficacy of the social role models (Holloway, 1992; Morgan & Sprenkle, 2007). This model may not be inclusive enough to meet all of the supervisee's needs.

Authors' Preferred Selection of Supervision Models
from the Case Studies

Authors' Preferred Supervision Model for Case 1

Based on the supervisory question and case presentation, the microcounseling supervision model would be an excellent way to conduct this supervision session. Using the CIRF would assist the supervisee in better understanding the micro- and macrocounseling skills and even help her process her fears about being lost in the counseling session.

Chapter Seven Review

Basic Tenet

- Supervisees benefit from a standardized, atheoretical approach, assisting them in reviewing, offering feedback, and evaluating micro- and macrocounseling skills and the counseling interview.

When to Use

- When essential microskills are not effectively utilized, selecting the microcounseling supervision model is suggested.

Supervisor's Roles and Behaviors

- Use the Counselor Interview Rating Form (CIRF) as a mechanism for creating a reciprocal supervision process for offering constructive feedback.
- Choose from the three MSM components based upon supervisee's needs: Reviewing Skills with Intention, Classifying Skills with Mastery, and Processing Supervisory Needs.

Supervisor's Emphasis and Goals

- Assist the supervisee with clarifying and defining all micro- and macrocounseling skills.
- Identify and classify observed skills with intention using the CIRF.
- Process the strengths and liabilities of the counseling session, answering the supervisory question.

Limitations

- The major limitation is that MSM is best utilized when there is a videotape or digital tape of a counseling session. In some settings, obtaining a recording of a counseling session does not easily occur.

Authors' Preferred Supervision Model for Case 2

Based on the supervision question and the case presentation, interpersonal process recall (IPR) would be an excellent preferred choice for this supervision session. This model allows for safe yet gentle questions to explore and lead the supervisee's feelings, thoughts, and experiences about the counseling interaction. The skill of immediacy allows the supervisee to examine "what's occurring now during the counseling session."

Chapter Eight Review

Basic Tenet

- Supervisees need an environment where they can safely analyze their communication styles and strategies.

When to Use

- If a supervisee seems to be stuck in the counseling interview, this method allows for safe, immediate feedback and a chance to reflect on the counseling experience.

Supervisor's Roles and Behaviors

- Stop the videotape at any time to discuss essential personal and/or counseling issues. If a videotape is not available, lead the supervision session with needed questions.

Supervisor's Emphasis and Goals

- The main goal is to stop a counseling videotape or supervisory session and use the skill of immediacy to gently discover counseling blocks, styles, and experiences.

Limitations

- This supervision approach is best used with video or digital recordings, so the supervisor can start and stop the interview when processing is required. However a variation of IPR can be used without recordings by asking the supervisee to recall how he or she felt at that moment.

Authors' Preferred Supervision Model for Case 3

Based on the supervision question and the case presentation, any developmental model would serve the supervisee well. Using the Stoltenberg, McNeil, and Delworth developmental supervision model, the first supervisory task would be an assessment of the supervisee's developmental level. In this case, the supervision questions direct the supervisor to level 2. This shows the supervisee moving toward independence yet needing encouragement from the supervisor. The growth areas needing attention may be interventions, skill competency, and client conceptualization.

Chapter Four Review

Basic Tenet

- According to the Stoltenberg, McNeil, and Delworth developmental supervision model, supervisees grow at individual paces, with differing needs and styles of learning and often with stages of growth that are dependent upon skill level and need of the client.

When to Use

- Use this model when assessment of the developmental level of the supervisee is needed and surmised.

Supervisor's Emphasis and Goals

- Assess the supervisee's developmental level of functioning from levels 1 through 4
- Understand the supervisee's world, motivational levels, and degree of autonomy
- Identify needed growth areas in each of the four levels, using the nine intervention areas listed below.

Supervisee Growth Areas

- Interventions
- Skill competence
- Assessment techniques
- Interpersonal assessment
- Client conceptualization
- Individual differences
- Theoretical orientation
- Treatment goals and plans
- Professional ethics

Limitations

This model does not go deep enough into specific supervision methods for each supervisee level, and it focuses only on student development as supervisees (Haynes, Corey, & Moulton, 2003).

Authors' Preferred Supervision Model for Case 4

Based on the supervision questions and the case presentation, a theoretical specific model of supervision may be the best fit. In this case, a family systems Bowenian supervision model would be demonstrated within the supervisory session.

Chapter Five Review

Basic Tenet

- The basic tenet of Bowen's generational family systems supervision model stresses the importance of the emotional system of the family unit.

When to Use

- Use this approach when the supervisee needs to better understand his client, not in isolation, but within the entire family system.

Supervisor's Roles and Behavior

- The supervisor may work on the main constructs of the supervision sessions using correlating counseling techniques such as genograms, triangulation, and differentiation.
- The supervisor acts as a teacher and coach.

Supervisor's Emphasis and Goals

- The main goal is to understand how the client reacts and responds within an entire family system.

Supervisee Growth Areas

- The supervisee will learn personal and client areas of family dysfunction and possible relationships needing healing.

Limitations

- This supervision model may address the client's and supervisee's family system, but it may not address the personal needs of the client.

Authors' Preferred Supervision Model for Case 5

Based on the supervision questions and the case presentation, the social roles supervision models provide an effective strategy. Using the discrimination supervision model would assist the supervisee in answering her concerns and questions. In this case, the supervisee is requesting assistance focusing on the process and conceptualization of the counseling session. The supervisor's role would be that of teacher and counselor.

Chapter Six Review

Basic Tenet

- Supervisees benefit from those supervisors who work from multiple theoretical orientations and focus on supervisee's needs by being able to respond flexibly with any needed strategy, technique, and/or guidance based upon the supervisor's role and focus.

When to Use

- When the supervisee is unaware of her own experience with clients, the discrimination model assists in expanding counseling knowledge base.

Supervisor's Roles and Behaviors

- The supervisor responds flexibly with needed role of teacher, counselor, and/or consultant.
- The supervisor selects the necessary focus.

Supervisor's Emphasis and Goals

- Emphasize two primary functions during each supervision session, that of the supervisors's role and focus.
- Three supervisor roles selected based upon supervisee needs are teacher, counselor, and consultant.
- Each of these roles has three areas of focus for skill-building purposes.
- The three areas of focus are process, conceptualization, and personalization.

Limitations

- There is limited empirical evidence testing the efficacy of the social role models (Holloway, 1992; Morgan & Sprenkle, 2007). This model may not be inclusive enough to meet all of the supervisee's needs.

Index

Note: Page numbers followed by a f indicate a figure; followed by a t indicate a table.